What a Young Woman Ought to Know

Mary Wood-Allen

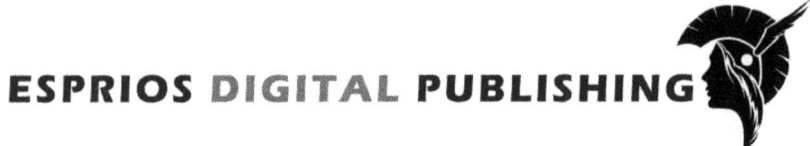

Commendations
from Eminent
Men & Women

*What
A Young Woman
Ought to Know*

COMMENDED BY REV. F.B. MEYER
The Eminent English Preacher and Author

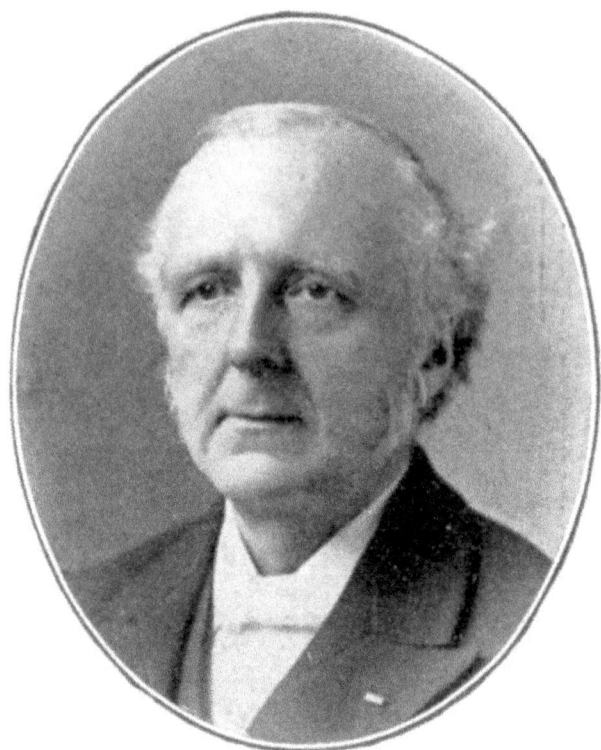

REV. F.B. MEYER, B.A.

Minister of Christ Church, Westminster, London,
Author of "Israel, A Prince with
God," "Elijah; Tried by Fire," "The
Bells of Is," etc., etc.

"The questions which are dealt with in the 'Self and Sex Series' of books are always being asked, and if the answer is not forthcoming from pure and wise lips it will be obtained through vicious and empirical channels. I therefore greatly commend this series of books, which are written lucidly and purely, and will afford the necessary information without pandering to unholy and sensual passion. I should like to see a wide and judicious distribution of this literature among Christian circles."

COMMENDED BY CHARLES M. SHELDON
The Eminent American Preacher and Author

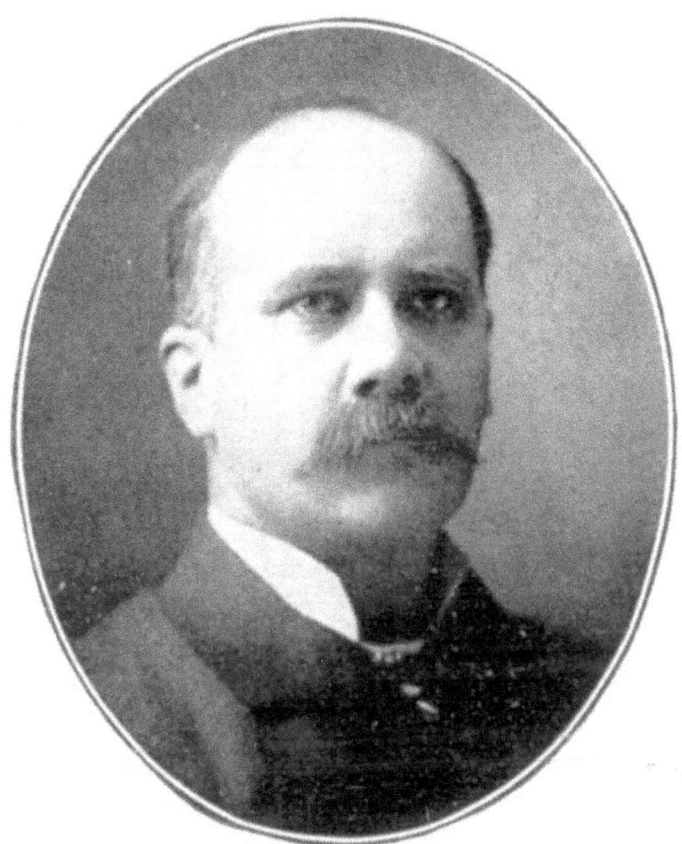

CHARLES M. SHELDON, D.D.

Pastor of Central Congregational Church,
Topeka, Kansas; author of "In His Steps,"
"The Crucifixion of Philip Strong,"
"Lend a Hand," "Born to Serve."

"It is a pleasure to call attention to the books of the 'Self and Sex Series' which have been prepared with great wisdom for the express purpose of teaching the truth concerning the subjects which are painfully neglected."

COMMENDED BY MRS. M.W. SEWALL
The Eminent American Educator

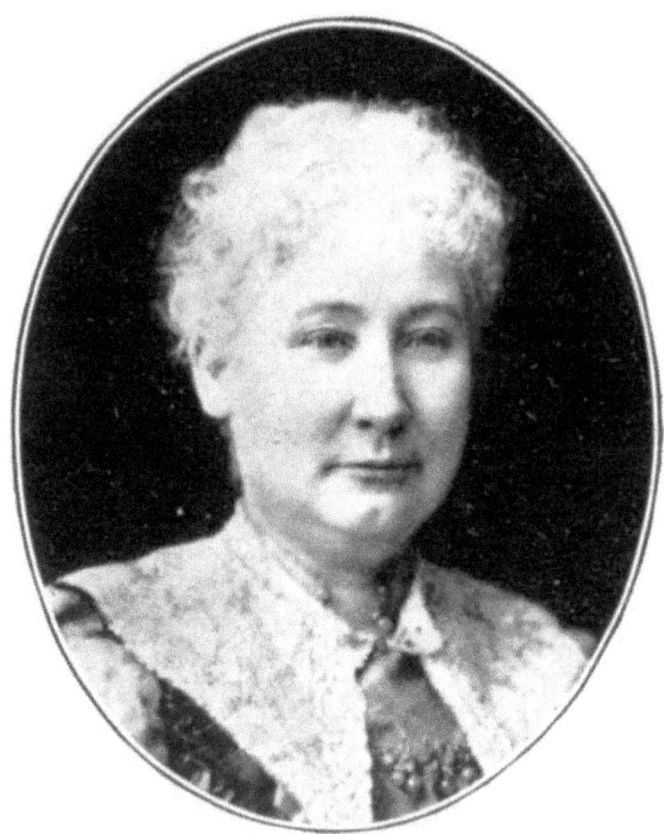

MRS. MAY WRIGHT SEWALL

Principal of the Girls' Classical School;
former President of the International Council
of Women; and Nominee of the International
Congress of Women.

"I am profoundly grateful that a subject of such information to young women should be treated in a manner at once so noble and so delicate that any pure-minded teacher or mother may read or discuss its pages with young girls without the slightest chance of wounding the most delicate sensibilities, or by being misunderstood."

COMMENDED BY MRS. M.L. DICKINSON
The Eminent American Christian Worker

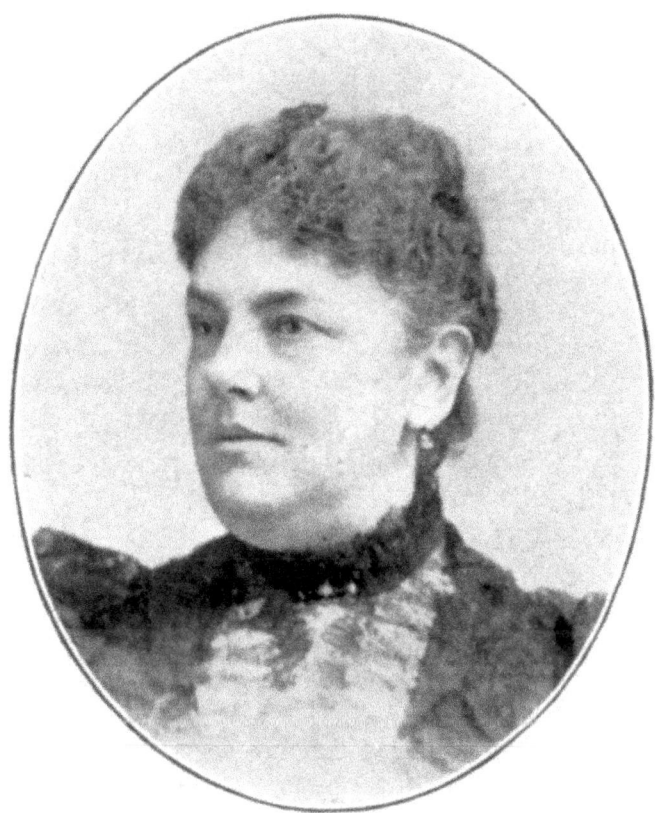

MRS. MARY LOWE DICKINSON

Former President of the National Council of Women;
General Secretary of the Order of The King's
Daughters; Emeritus Professor of Literature
Denver University; Editor of "The Silver Cross;"
Author of "The Temptation of Katharine
Gray," "One Little Life," etc., etc.

"Any young woman, knowing all that this volume teaches, has an essential foundation for whatever other knowledge she may acquire."

COMMENDED BY MRS. M.B. CARSE
The Eminent American Christian Worker

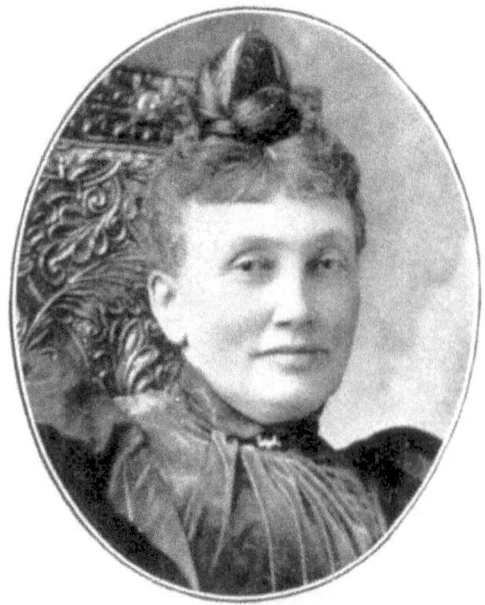

MRS. MATILDA B. CARSE

Founder of the Woman's Temple, Chicago.

"As a mother, I can truly say that my heart goes out to you in endorsement of this book. It is pure and instructive on the delicate subjects that mean so much to our daughters, to their future as home-keepers, wives and mothers, and to the future generations. It can but create a more reverent ideal of life in every girl who reads it, and I wish every daughter in the land could reap of its benefit."

COMMENDED BY MRS. E.C. STANTON
The Eminent American Lecturer and Author

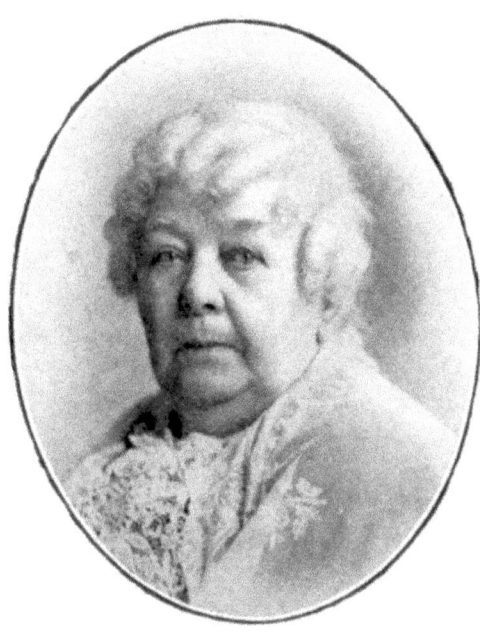

MRS. ELIZABETH CADY STANTON

Noted Woman Suffragist, Lecturer
and Author.

"Your books I consider a valuable addition to the literature of the day on social ethics. The many facts you state are not only important for a knowledge of social science, but involve good health and morals."

COMMENDED BY MR. C.N. CRITTENTON
The Eminent American Philanthropist

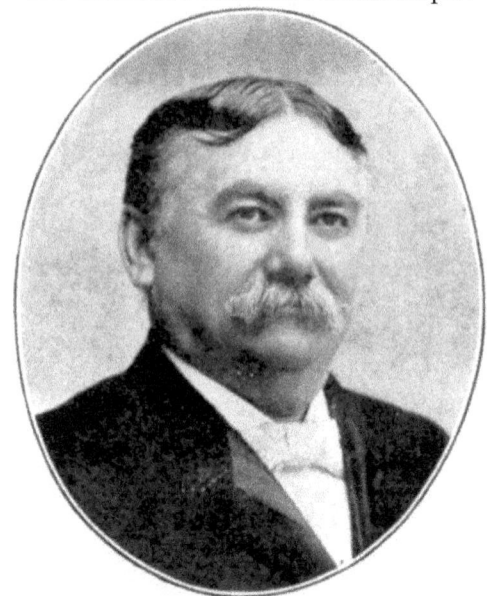

CHARLES N. CRITTENTON

Founder of the National Florence Crittenton Mission

"The frequent excuse which parents give for not enlightening their children on these most important points is that they have never known how to do so. This excuse can no longer be considered valid.

"Dr. Wood-Allen has a remarkable gift in the facility and refinement with which she is able to approach the most delicate subject without arousing a single morbid and sensitive impulse."

COMMENDED BY MRS. H. CAMPBELL
The Eminent American Author and Educator

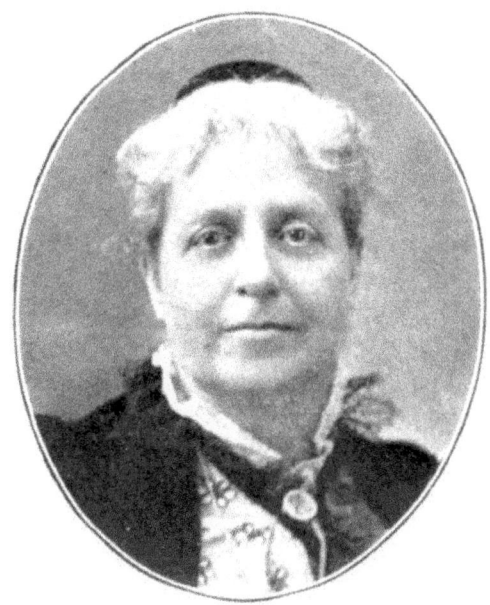

MRS. HELEN CAMPBELL

Dean of the Department of Household Economics in the Kansas State Agricultural College. Author of "Prisoners of Poverty," "Wage Earners," etc., etc.

"I cannot speak too warmly of your invaluable series. There is hardly a woman in America so thoroughly qualified by education, long experience, deep sympathies, and, most excellent of all gifts, as deep common sense, as Dr. Mary Wood-Allen, to meet the growing need, or rather the growing sense of need. Mothers and fathers alike will be helped and enlightened by these simple, clear-phrased, wholesome books, and they deserve all the success already their own."

COMMENDED BY L.M.N. STEVENS
The Eminent Temperance Worker

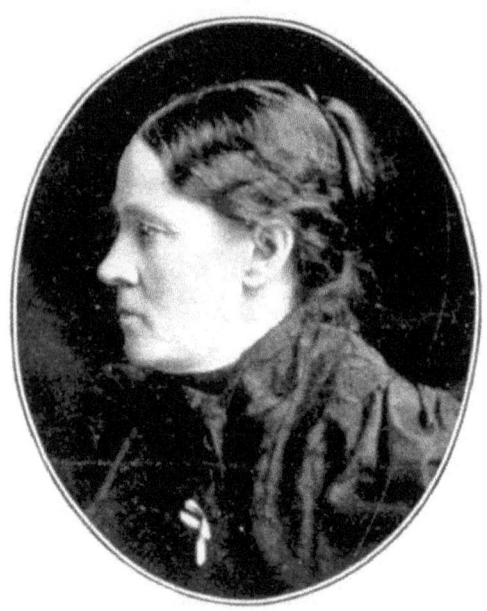

MRS. LILLIAN M.N. STEVENS

President of National Woman's Christian
Temperance Union.

"I consider the book 'What a Young Wife Ought to Know' a wise and safe teacher. It is a careful and delicate presentation of vital truths which have to do with the happiness and welfare of home life."

COMMENDED BY EMINENT AMERICAN AUTHORS AND EDITORS

MARGARET WARNER MORLEY

Author of "The Song of Life," "Life and Love," "The Bee People," etc.

"There is an awful need for the book, and it does what it has undertaken to do better than anything of the kind I have ever read. You may rely upon me to make it known wherever I can."

ELISABETH ROBINSON SCOVIL

Superintendent of the Newport Hospital, and Associate Editor of the Ladies' Home Journal; Author of "The Care of Children," etc.

"'What a Young Woman Ought to Know' is characterized by purity of tone and delicacy of treatment.

"It is one which a mother can place with confidence in the hands of her daughter. Reverent knowledge is the surest safeguard of innocence, and it is every mother's duty to see that the young girl committed to her charge is duly forearmed by being forewarned of the dangers that lie around her."

Pure Books on Avoided Subjects

Books for Men

By Sylvanus Stall, D.D.

"What a Young Boy Ought to Know."
"What a Young Man Ought to Know."
"What a Young Husband Ought to Know."
"What a Man of 45 Ought to Know."

Books for Women

By Mrs. Mary Wood-Allen, M.D.
And Mrs. Emma F.A. Drake, M.D.

"What a Young Girl Ought to Know."
"What a Young Woman Ought to Know."
"What a Young Wife Ought to Know."
"What a Woman of 45 Ought to Know."

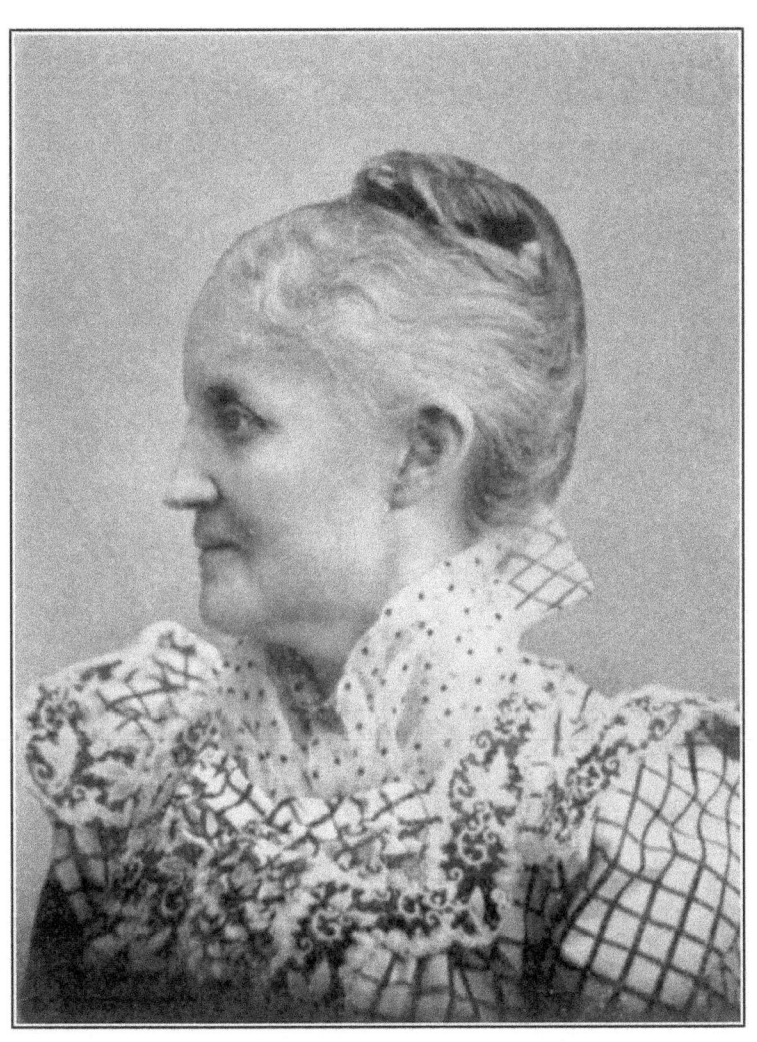

MRS. MARY WOOD-ALLEN, M.D.

NEW REVISED EDITION

Self and Sex Series

*What
A Young Woman
Ought to Know*

BY

MRS. MARY WOOD-ALLEN, M.D.

National Superintendent of the Purity Department Woman's Christian Temperance Union; Author of "What a Young Girl Ought to Know," "Marvels of Our Bodily Dwelling," "Child Confidence Rewarded," "Teaching Truth," "Almost a Man," "Almost a Woman."

1889

TO
THE DAUGHTER DEAR,
WHOSE INTIMATE AND CONFIDENTIAL COMPANIONSHIP
FROM
CHILDHOOD TO WOMANHOOD HAS MADE IT POSSIBLE
FOR ME TO FEEL A SYMPATHETIC INTEREST IN
THE LIFE-PROBLEMS OF ALL GIRLS, THIS
BOOK IS MOST LOVINGLY
DEDICATED
BY HER
MOTHER

CONTENTS.

PART I.
CHAPTER I.
WHAT ARE YOU WORTH?

The first great lesson to learn, your own importance — Probably twelve million young women in the United States — What it means for one of them to be sick — Woman's work in the world — The using of spiritual forces — How much are you worth to your home, to the community, to the state, to the nation, to the race?

CHAPTER II.
CARE OF BODY.

Your body is your dwelling — It expresses you — We can judge of character by the external appearance — The body also an instrument and should be taken care of — Not "fussy" to take care of it in youth — We should prepare for life

CHAPTER III.
FOOD.

A desire for health creates a desire to know how to obtain it — The question of diet — We eat to repair waste and to supply new material — Overstudy less a cause of illness than wrong eating — Tea and coffee not foods — Alcoholic beverages interfere with digestion — Dyspepsia produced by worry — We should give ourselves to our friends — Young women should study scientific cookery

CHAPTER IV.
SLEEP.

Every thought, activity, or motion causes expenditure of force — In sleep the energy restored — Amount of sleep needed — Effect of sleeplessness — Causes of unrefreshing sleep — Ventilation of sleeping rooms — Beauty sleep

CHAPTER V.
BREATHING.

How often we breathe — What is accomplished by breathing — Office of oxygen in the blood — Breathing our measure of ability — Breathing gymnastics, their value — Importance of the diaphragm in breathing

CHAPTER VI.
HINDRANCES TO BREATHING.

Effect of sitting attitudes — How to counteract this — Wrong positions in standing — Restrictions of clothing — Rule for the tightness of clothing — Why tight dresses may feel comfortable

CHAPTER VII.
ADDED INJURIES FROM TIGHT CLOTHING.

The effect upon the heart — Danger of exercising in tight dress — Effect of tight clothing upon the kidneys, upon the liver, stomach, and bowels — How the bowels are held in the abdomen — Influence of tight clothing upon the pelvic organs — Upon the circulation — A tapering waist a deformity

CHAPTER VIII.
EXERCISE.

The purpose of physical culture — Balance between waste and supply — Gymnastic dress a necessity — Value of housework — Bicycle riding — Dancing — Skating — Lawn tennis — Running up and down stairs — Bathing

CHAPTER IX.
BATHING.

Beauty of complexion — Condition of skin indicates condition of digestive organs — Pimples — Constipation — Thermal bath — Foot bath — Time to bathe — Daily baths — The use of soaps — Wrinkles — Care of the hands

PART II.
CHAPTER X.
CREATIVE POWER.

We have Godlike powers: reason, imagination, conferring life — Organs of individual life same in both sexes — Differences between the sexes in size — Dignity of man

CHAPTER XI.
BUILDING BRAINS.

Babies born deaf, dumb, blind and helpless — The activities of the baby build its brains — Our brains develop through cultivation of the senses — Certain areas of brain govern certain movements of body — Can learn how to build up any part of brain — Professor Gates' experiments in training dogs — Creation of habits — Effects of malevolent passions, such as anger, worry, etc.

CHAPTER XII.
YOU ARE MORE THAN BODY OR MIND.

You are neither body nor mind, you are spirit — Your relationship to God — God's obligation to us — Our obligation to Him — God's school — His method of teaching us.

CHAPTER XIII.
SPECIAL PHYSIOLOGY.

Differences between boys and girls — Boys need our sympathy — The crisis in the girl's life — Sex in mind — Description of the sex organs

CHAPTER XIV.
BECOMING A WOMAN.

All life from an egg — The human egg — Menstruation — Girls may injure themselves through ignorance — Value of sex.

CHAPTER XV.
ARTIFICIALITIES OF CIVILIZED LIFE.

Menstruation should be painless — Dr. Mary Jacobi's opinion — Dr. Emmett on the artificial life of young women.

CHAPTER XVI.
SOME CAUSES OF PAINFUL MENSTRUATION.

Woman not necessarily a semi-invalid — Effects of wrong clothing on the young girl — Evils of novel reading — Evils of constipation — Congestions produced by displacements — Serious results of abdominal displacements — Value of abdominal bandage — How to make one — How to wear it — Effects of wrong attitude — Standing on one foot — Correct attitude.

CHAPTER XVII.
FEMALE DISEASES.

Displacements of uterus — Leucorrhea — Patent medicines — Honest physicians — Sitz baths for reducing congestions — Age at which menstruation first appears — Non-menstruation and consumption — Mechanical hindrances to menstruation — Suppression — Scanty flow — Profuse flow — Treatment.

CHAPTER XVIII.
CARE DURING MENSTRUATION.

No long walks or rides — May pursue usual avocations — If pain, keep quiet — Do not use alcoholics of any kind — Use of heat — Use of cold — Should you bathe at this time — Arrangement of clothing and napkins — Mental serenity.

CHAPTER XIX.
SOLITARY VICE.

Its results — Causes — Lack of cleanliness — Pin-worms — All functions attended with pleasure — Sex not low — Its development accompanied by increased power — How overcome the bad habit? — Remove causes of pelvic congestions — Train the senses — Study clouds, leaves, shapes, birds, etc.

CHAPTER XX.
BE GOOD TO YOURSELF.

What is real fun — The effects of a wrong idea of fun — Flirtations — Familiarities — Criticism of girls by young men — Class of girls who are most respected — Responsibility of girls — The conduct of a pure woman the safeguard of man.

CHAPTER XXI.
FRIENDSHIP BETWEEN BOYS AND GIRLS.

The meaning of friendship — Mother the girl's wisest confidante — Kissing — Friendship between brothers and sisters — Platonic friendships — The value of noble companionship.

CHAPTER XXII.
FRIENDSHIP BETWEEN GIRLS.

Gushing girls — Manly friendships — The highest type of friendship — To love truly is to grow strong by true giving.

CHAPTER XXIII.
EXERCISES.

Correct dressing — To overcome curvature — Round shoulders — To strengthen the back — To develop the chest — Abdominal muscles — To restore displaced organs.

CHAPTER XXIV.
RECREATIONS.

Walking — Running — Riding — Skating — Rowing — Cycling — Tennis — Swimming — Skipping — Dancing — Card-playing — Theatre-going.

PART III.
CHAPTER XXV.
LOVE.

Different ideas of different people — Much that is called love is selfishness — Love at first sight — Present conditions of society unnatural — Parents unwilling to teach their children, yet permit flirtations, etc. — What is love? — One word to express different phases of regard — Love of man and woman — Love should include mental congeniality, spiritual sympathy and physical attraction — Young people should have opportunity to get acquainted — Comradeship of young people — Love is a growth.

CHAPTER XXVI.
RESPONSIBILITY IN MARRIAGE.

Who is the young man? — What are his antecedents, his talents, his habits? — What sort of a family does he belong to? — The wife marries her husband's family — Girls should know this — A mother's privilege.

CHAPTER XXVII.
THE LAW OF HEREDITY.

A strange will — Should study the law of inheritance — Plant heredity — Race heredity — National characteristics — Individual inheritance — We are composite photographs — The law of heredity a beneficial law — Transmission of evil a warning — Bad tempers inherited — Atavism.

CHAPTER XXVIII.
HEREDITARY EFFECTS OF ALCOHOL, TOBACCO, ETC.

Alcoholism produces nerve degeneration — Tight lacing may have the same result — Nerve degeneracy may lead to alcoholism — Idiocy and inebriety increasing — Effects of wine — Evils of patent medicines — Inebriety of parents entails injury on offspring — Folly of marrying a man to reform him — Hereditary effects of morphine, chloral, etc. — Dangers of the tobacco habit — Inherited effects of tobacco.

CHAPTER XXIX.
FFECTS OF IMMORALITY ON THE RACE.

The law of God not a double law — The inherited effects of immorality — Millions die annually from its effects — Transmitted to child or wife — Contamination through a kiss.

CHAPTER XXX.
THE GOSPEL OF HEREDITY.

Inheritance of good so universal that we fail to think of it — Mercy shown to thousands of generations — Heredity not fatality — Effects of education transmitted — Experiments of Professor Gates on dogs — A divine inheritance.

CHAPTER XXXI.
REQUISITES OF A HUSBAND.

What is the young man's inheritance? — What are his ideas? — What is his estimate of woman? — What are his defects? — Are there adequate reasons why some should not marry? — May not married people be happy without children — A girl should know something of the personal habits of her future husband — Should consider her own personal habits — How freely may young people talk together?

CHAPTER XXXII.
ENGAGEMENTS.

Becoming engaged for fun — May not engaged young people throw aside restrictions? — Long engagements — The benefits of an engagement — Evils of a long engagement — Engagement a time of preparation — Sexual attraction not limited to local expression — Duty of the engaged young woman to her own family — Jealousy the quintessence of selfishness — Trust a suggestion to be true — Common sense needed in marriage — Hold your lover to the highest ideals.

CHAPTER XXXIII.
THE WEDDING.

Folly of preparing an elaborate trousseau — The way of one sensible girl — The wedding gifts — Bridal tours — The realities of wedded life.

PREFACE.

During a number of years it has been my privilege to be the confidante and counsellor of a large number of young women of various stations in life and in all parts of the United States.

These girls have talked freely with me concerning their plans, aspirations, fears and personal problems. It has been a great revelation to me to note with what unanimity they ask certain questions concerning conduct—queries which perhaps might astonish the mothers of those same girls, as they, doubtless, take it for granted that their daughters intuitively understand these fundamental laws of propriety.

The truth is that many girls who have been taught in the "ologies" of the schools, who have been trained in the conventionalities of society, have been left to pick up as they may their ideas upon personal conduct, and, coming face to face with puzzling problems, are at a loss, and perhaps are led into wrong ways of thinking and questionable ways of doing because no one has foreseen their dilemma and warned them how to meet it.

The subjects treated in this little book are discussed because every one of them has been the substance of a query propounded by some girl otherwise intelligent and well informed. They have been treated plainly and simply because they purport to be the frank conferences of a mother and daughter, between whom there can be no need of hesitation in dealing frankly with any question bearing on the life, health or happiness of the girl. There is therefore no need of apology; the book is its own excuse for being, the queries of the young women demand honest answers.

Life will be safer for the girl who understands her own nature and reverences her womanhood, who realizes her responsibility towards the human race and conducts herself in accordance with that realization.

Life will be nobler and purer in its possession and its transmission, if, from childhood onward to old age, the thought has been held that

"Life is a gift of God and is divine," and its physical is no less sacred than its mental or moral manifestation; if it has been understood that the foundations of character are laid in the habits formed in youth, and that a noble girlhood assures a grand maturity.

Dear girls who read this book, the mother-heart has gone out to you with great tenderness with every line herein written, with many an unspoken prayer that you will be helped, uplifted, inspired by its reading, and made more and more to feel

> "A sacred burden is this life ye bear.
> Look on it, lift it, bear it solemnly;
> Stand up and walk beneath it steadfastly;
> Fail not for sorrow, falter not for sin,
> But onward, upward, till the goal ye win."

Mary Wood-Allen.

ANN ARBOR, MICHIGAN.

PART I.
THE VALUE OF HEALTH, AND RESPONSIBILITY IN MAINTAINING IT.

CHAPTER I.

WHAT ARE YOU WORTH?

My Daughter Dear:

When I see you with your young girl friends, when I look into your bright faces and listen to your merry laughter and your girlish chatter, I wonder if any one of you understands how much you are worth. Now you may say, "I haven't any money in the bank, I have no houses or land, I am worth nothing," but that would only be detailing what you possess. It is not what you possess but what you are that determines what you are worth. One may possess much wealth and be worth very little.

I was reading the other day that the first great lesson for a *young man* to learn, the first fact to realize, is that he is of some importance; that upon his wisdom, energy and faithfulness all else depends, and that the world cannot get along without him. Now if this is true of young men, I do not see why it is not equally true of young women.

It is not after you have grown old that you will be of value to the world; it is now, in your young days, while you are laying the foundation of your character, that you are of great importance. We cannot say that the foundation is of no importance until the building is erected, for upon the right placing of the foundation depends the firmness and stability of the superstructure. Dr. Conwell, in his little book, "Manhood's Morning," estimates that there are twelve million young men in the United States between fourteen and twenty-eight years of age; that these twelve million young men represent latent physical force enough to dig the iron ore from the mines, manufacture it into wire, lay the foundation and construct completely the great Brooklyn Bridge in three hours; that they represent force enough, if rightly utilized, to dig the clay from the earth, manufacture the bricks and construct the great Chinese Wall in five days. If each one were to build himself a house twenty-five feet wide, these houses would line both sides of eight streets reaching across the continent from the Atlantic to the Pacific. For each one to be sick one day is equal to thirty thousand being sick an entire year.

Now, if there are twelve million young men in the United States, we may estimate that there are an equal number of young women. Although we cannot calculate accurately the amount of physical force represented by these young women, there are some things we can tell. We know that for each one of these young women to be sick one day means thirty thousand sick one year. Just imagine the loss to the country, and the gain to posterity if it can be prevented!

Rome endeavored to create good soldiery, but was not able to produce strength and courage through physical culture of the men alone. Not until she began the physical education of the women, the young women, was she able to insure to the nation a race of strong, hardy, vigorous soldiery. So the health of the young women of to-day is of great importance to the nation, for upon their vigor and soundness of body depend to a very great extent the health and capacity of future generations. We are told that in the State of Massachusetts, in one year, there were lost twenty-eight thousand five hundred (28,500) years of time through the illness of working-people by preventable diseases. Dr. Buck, in his "Hygiene," tells us that one hundred thousand persons die every year through preventable diseases, that one hundred and fifty thousand are constantly sick through preventable diseases, and that the loss to the nation, through the illness of working-people by diseases that might have been prevented, is more than a hundred million dollars a year. So we can see that each individual has a pecuniary value to the nation. You are worth just as much to the nation as you can earn. If you earn a dollar a day, you are not only worth a dollar a day to yourself and to your personal employer, but you are worth a dollar a day to the nation; and if, through illness, you are laid aside for one day, the nation, as well as yourself, is pecuniarily the loser.

Young women could not build the houses that would line eight streets from New York to San Francisco, but, rightly educated, they could convert each one of these houses into a home, and to found a home and conduct it properly is to help the world. It is so easy to measure what is done with physical strength. We can see what men are doing when they build railroads, construct immense bridges and towering buildings, but it is more difficult to measure what is done through intellectual and spiritual forces; and woman's work in the world is not so much the using of strength as it is the using of those finer forces which go to build up men and women. With this thought in your mind, can you answer the question, How much are you worth? How much are you worth to yourself? How much are you worth in your home? How much money would your parents be willing to accept in place of yourself? How much are you worth to the community in which you live? How much are you worth to the state, the nation, the human race?

You can recognize your value in the home when you remember how much you are the center of all that goes on there, how much your interest is consulted in everything that is done by father and mother. You can realize your value to the state when you realize how much money is spent for the education of young people, how cultured men and women give the best of their lives to your instruction. You cannot measure your value to the human race until you begin to think that the young people of to-day are creating the condition of the world in fifty or one hundred years to come; that you, through your physical health, or lack of it, are to become a source of strength or weakness in future years, if you are a mother. It is all right that young women should think of marriage and motherhood, provided they think of it in the right way.

I want you to reverence yourself, to realize your own importance, to feel that you are a necessity to God's perfect plan. When we are young and feel that we are of no account in the world, it is difficult to realize that God's complete plan cannot be carried out without us. The smallest, tiniest rivet or bolt may be of such great importance in the construction of an engine that its loss means the incapacity of that piece of machinery to do its work. As God has placed you in the world, He has placed you here to do a specific work for Him and for humanity, and your failure to do that work means the failure of His complete and perfect plan. Now can you begin to see how much you are worth? And can you begin to realize that in the conduct of your life as a young woman you are a factor of immense importance to the great problem of the evolution of the human race? In the light of these thoughts I would like to have you ask yourself this question every day, How much am I worth?

CHAPTER II.

CARE OF BODY.

The question "How much are you worth?" is not answered by discussing your bodily conditions, for your body is not yourself. It is your dwelling, but not you. It, however, expresses you.

A man builds a house, and through it expresses himself. The external appearance causes the observer to form an opinion of him, and each apartment bears the impress of his individuality. To look at the house and then to walk through it will tell you much of the man. The outside will tell you whether he is neat, orderly and artistic, or whether he cares nothing for the elements of beauty and neatness. If you go into his parlor, you can judge whether he cares most for show or for comfort. His library will reveal to you the character of his mind, and the dining-room will indicate by its furnishings and its viands whether he loves the pleasures of sense more than health of body. You do not need to see the man to have a pretty clear idea of him.

So the body is our house, and our individuality permeates every part of it. Those who look at our bodily dwelling can gain a very good idea of what we are. The external appearance will indicate to a great extent our character. We glance at one man and say, "He is gross, sensual, cruel, domineering;" at another and say, "He is intellectual, spiritual, fine-grained, benevolent." So we judge of entire strangers, and usually find the character largely corresponds to our judgment, if, later, we come to know the person.

The anatomist and microscopist who penetrates into the secrets of his bodily house after the inhabitant has moved out can tell much of his habits, his thoughts, his capacities and powers by the traces of himself which he has left on the insensate walls of his dwelling. The care of the body, then, adds to our value, because it gives us a better instrument, a better medium of expression.

The old saying, "A workman is known by his tools," is equally true of the body. The carpenter who cares for his saws, chisels and planes, who keeps them sharp and free from rust, will be able to do better work than the one who carelessly allows them to become nicked, broken, handleless or rusted. The finer the work which one does, the greater the care he must take of the instruments with which he works. A jack-knife will do to whittle a pine stick, but the carver of intricate designs must have his various sharp tools with which to make the delicate lines and tracings.

When we speak of health and physical conditions in discussing the question of your value, we are discussing the instrument upon whose integrity depends your ability to demonstrate your value.

Many young people think it nonsense to pay attention to the preservation of health. I have heard them say, "O, I don't want to be so fussy! It will do for old folks to be coddling themselves, but I want a good time. I'd rather die ten years sooner and have some fun while I do live."

I wonder what these same young people would think if they should hear a workman say, "Well, I have here a fine kit of tools; I am assured that if they are destroyed they will never be replaced; but now, while I am learning my trade, I don't want to be 'so fussy' about keeping them in order. It will do for 'boss workmen' to take care of everything so constantly, but now I want to break stones with these delicate hammers, to cut nails with these razor-bladed knives, to crack nuts with these slender pincers. By and by, when I am older, I'll use them as they should be used, but I think it's all nonsense to be so careful now." If in later years you should hear him complain that he had nothing to work with, would you feel like pitying him?

No "kit of tools" was ever so complete as is the bodily instrument given to each one of us. Its mechanism has been the inspiration of inventors; it combines all forms of mechanical devices; its delicacy, intricacy, completeness and adaptability challenge the admiration of the philosopher, the engineer, the master mechanic.

I cannot here tell you of all its wonders,[1] but I would like to give you such an exalted idea of its importance that you would look upon it with reverence and take a justifiable pride in keeping it in perfect working order. I would like to make you feel your personal responsibility in regard to its condition.

You know that in the ages past men believed the body to be the individual, and they endeavored through care of the body to build up mental as well as physical power. In those days the acrobat and the sage were found working side by side in the gymnasium, the one to gain physical strength, the other to increase his mental ability, and each profited as he desired.

When men made the discovery that the body is not the individual, but merely his dwelling and instrument of expression, they came to feel less regard for it, and lost their interest in its care and culture. Even the early Christians, forgetting what Paul said about the body as a temple, began to call it vile, and thought it an evidence of great piety to treat it with contempt. I have read of one religious sect who believed that the Creator of the body could not have been the Creator of the soul, and held that the chief object of God's government was to deliver the captive souls of men from their bodily prisons.

When men began to understand that the thinking principle was the real self and the body merely a material encasement, it was no wonder that they valued the body less and held mind as of great value. They failed to see that mind without a material organ of expression is, in this world, of no account. A great pianist with no piano could not make music, and he would be considered a strange being if he did not care for his instrument most scrupulously. Think of a Rubinstein voluntarily breaking the piano strings or smashing the keys, while he made discordant poundings, and excusing himself by saying that it was "fussy" to take care of a piano until it was old. You cannot imagine such a thing. We can all appreciate the value of a man-made instrument or machine; but the God-created body, a combination of machines and instruments of marvelous power and delicacy, we neglect or treat with absolute, positive injury, and excuse ourselves on the ground that when it is old we will treat it more kindly.

Melville says it is a sin to die, ignoring what is to be done with the body. "That body," he says, "has been redeemed, that body has been appointed to a glorious condition."

It seems to me we prize the body far more after its use for us is at an end than while it is ours to use. We do not neglect the dead; we dress them in beautiful garments, we adorn them with flowers, we follow them to the grave with religious ceremonies, we build costly monuments to place over their graves, and then we go to weep over their last resting-place.

After all, is it not life that we should value? Life here and hereafter, not death, is the real thing for which we should prepare, and earthly life without a sound body is not life full and complete. Life is joy, vigor, elasticity, freedom from pain or illness, enjoyment of all innocent pleasures in maturity as well as in youth. We have no right to look forward to decrepitude, to failure in zest of living, to lessening of real enjoyment because of coming years. Life should increase in beauty and usefulness, in ability and joyousness, as the years bring us a wider experience, and this will be the case if we in youth have been wise enough to lay the foundation of health by a wise, thoughtful, prudent care of our bodies and our minds.

FOOTNOTES:

[1] This Dr. Mary Wood-Allen has done in a volume entitled "Marvels of Our Bodily Dwelling." This book teaches physiology and hygiene, by metaphor, parable, and allegory in a most charming way. Superbly illustrated. 12mo. Price, cloth, $1.50, post free.

CHAPTER III.

FOOD.

If I can arouse in your mind a most earnest desire to be strong and vigorous, I shall not find it necessary to give you very minute directions, for if you have the ambition you will find the way. If I could excite in you an intense longing to visit Paris, I should know that you would begin to seek for the way of getting there. If I could create in you an earnest aspiration to be well and physically strong, I should know that you would seek for the books that would give you the necessary instruction. It will not be needful to talk of rules and restrictions if I can make you feel the glory of having a sound body.

If you were starting on a journey, I should not need to warn you of by-paths, of traps, or of dangers if I could be assured that your eye was fixed upon your ultimate destination. So it is in the matter of health; and yet there are some general rules or principles which I might lay down for your consideration.

In regard to the matter of diet. I do not want you to be hampered by "don'ts" and restrictions as to what you shall eat, but I do want you to eat with the thought in view that eating is to be governed by judgment and not by the pleasures of sense. Why do we eat? Not merely because the food tastes good. There is a better reason. We eat to live. We know that the food which we take into our bodies is digested, elaborated and assimilated—that is, made over into ourselves—and unless this digestion, elaboration and assimilation is properly conducted, we shall not be fully and completely nourished. Our body is made up of cells; the food which we eat is transformed into cell structure, and this new cell-material takes the place of the worn-out cells. Our reason would tell us that if too little material is furnished, cells will not be properly repaired and ill-health will follow. Our reason would tell us in the same way that if too much material is furnished, the machine will be clogged and the work will not be properly done. We will also understand at once that an irregular supply of new material would interfere with the elaboration of that which is undergoing the process of digestion and assimilation. We can see, too, that unless the various tissues receive the material which they can transform into themselves, they will not be fully repaired. If material is taken into the system which supplies no tissue with what it needs, this material becomes a source of irritation.

These general rules borne in mind are sufficient to guide us into a wiser life than if we do not understand them; and, understanding these general principles, we will be anxious to study the particular rules which govern digestion and assimilation.

I have known young women in college to be so absolutely ignorant or indifferent to physiological law as to be injuring themselves constantly by disobedience of such laws. I knew one girl, supposed to be a very fine student, and to have brought on "fits" by overstudy, while away at school. I had an opportunity to investigate the case, and I discovered that she had been eating from morning till night. She carried nuts, and candy, and apples in her pocket, had pickles and cake in her room, and studied and munched until it was no doubt a disturbed digestion, rather than an overused brain, that caused the "fits."

If you will eat regularly of plain meat, vegetables, fruits, cereals, milk and eggs, plainly prepared, and avoid rich pastries, cakes, puddings, pickles and sweetmeats, you will have compassed the round of healthful diet, and need give yourself very little anxiety in regard to anything more. I should like to emphasize the fact, however, that tea and coffee are not foods. They are irritants, stimulants, nerve-poisons. They bring nothing to the system to build it up. They satisfy the sense of hunger without having contributed to the nourishment of the body. If you are wise you will avoid them. You will not create for yourself any false necessities. You will avoid the use of alcohol in all forms, whether wine, ales, beer or cider, as well as in the stronger forms, because you will know that these products interfere with digestion. Dr. Kellogg, of Battle Creek, has made an experiment which proved that sherry to the amount of 1 per cent. of the contents of the stomach retarded digestion nearly 4 per cent.

He calculates that 1 per cent. of sherry would be equal to two tenths of 1 per cent. of alcohol, and it would be necessary to take less than an ordinary tablespoonful of the wine to obtain this percentage.

When 3 per cent. of claret was used (equivalent to three-tenths of 1 per cent. of alcohol), there was marked diminution in digestive activity. This certainly proves that even the so-called light wines are injurious, and certainly the drinks that contain a large per cent. of alcohol must be that much more hurtful.

If you use good judgment both as to the quality and quantity of foods, you need then give the matter very little thought. People sometimes make themselves dyspeptics by worrying about what they eat. Eat what is set before you, making a judicious choice both as to variety and quantity, and then determine that your food shall digest.

When you live upon the higher plane of thought, you will not be so much interested in the question of food as regards gustatory pleasure. You will understand that eating is a necessity, but you will not be thinking about it; you will not be desiring to please the sense of taste; you will see that there are higher forms of sociability than mere eating with friends, and you will not be so interested in late suppers, and in various forms of sense gratification because you enjoy more thoroughly the higher pleasures. You will serve your friends with delicate food, simply and daintily prepared, and seasoned with that wit and wisdom which remain as a permanent mental pabulum. You will make them feel that when you come to visit them you come not to get something to eat, but to enjoy them, to receive from them the inspiration which they can give. We often treat our friends as if we thought they came as beggars for physical food. It is a much higher compliment to treat them as though we thought they came to exchange thoughts with us, to walk with us in the higher paths of living, and that the physical food we give them is only incidental. I was once entertained where a company of intelligent, cultured people were assembled, and we did not see the hostess from the time we entered the house until supper was served. She sat at the table, worried and anxious, and after the supper was over she did not make her appearance until just as we were about to leave. She did not pay us the high compliment of giving us herself, but she bestowed upon us that which a hired cook might have given.

You remember what Emerson says: "I pray you, O excellent wife, cumber not yourself and me to get a curiously rich dinner for this man and woman who have just alighted at our gate. These things, if they desire them, they can get for a few shillings at any village inn; but rather let that stranger see, if he will, in your looks, accents and behavior, your heart and earnestness, your thought and will, that which he cannot buy at any price in any city, and which he may travel miles and dine sparely and sleep hardly to behold."

It would indeed be worth your while to study food scientifically, to know how to prepare dainty and tempting dishes wholesomely, and then to serve your guests with such beauty of manner, such graciousness of courtesy, that they will remember the meal they have taken with you as idyllic in its simplicity, beauty and helpfulness.

CHAPTER IV.

SLEEP.

Shakespeare writes of "Sleep that knits up the ravelled sleeve of care." The metaphor is striking, but not accurate. To knit up that which is ravelled implies using the old material in repairing the damage, but that is not the way in which the body is rebuilt. The old material is thrown out and new material put in its place, and that largely takes place during sleep. We have read of brownies who came at night and swept and churned and baked while the housewife slept. So, in our bodily dwelling, the vital forces are our brownies, and they can work more uninterruptedly while we are asleep than when we are calling on them to move us from place to place, or to aid us in various activities.

Much of life's processes must remain a mystery to us, but certain things we have learned, and one is that perfect health cannot be maintained, strong nerves cannot be constructed, nor a clear brain be built without plenty of sleep. The baby sleeps almost continually because he is building so much new structure. The growing child needs more sleep than the adult; but even after reaching maturity sleep cannot be materially lessened without injury to the whole organization.

We appreciate the need of food. We are often very needlessly alarmed for fear that we shall starve from one meal to the next, but few of us realize that food cannot be assimilated, built into tissue, without some hours in which the vital forces can devote themselves wholly to the work of assimilation. During the working hours of the day we are expending force. The brain is using it in thought, the muscles are calling for force in various activities, the emotions are expending energy, and each of these activities is creating changes in the cells of the body. We know that life in the body is only possible through constant death of the atoms of which it is composed. We can only live because we are constantly dying. Huxley says, "For every vital act, life is used up. All work implies waste, and the work of life results directly or indirectly in the waste of protoplasm (which is the cell substance). Every word uttered by a speaker costs him some physical loss, and in the strictest sense he burns that others may have light."

Each word, thought, activity, emotion causes expenditure, and unless expenditure is in some way made good, there will be bankruptcy. How shall we get back the energy we have expended and so restore our vital forces to their equilibrium? The protoplasm of which our cells are made we can obtain from the protoplasm of animal and vegetable substances which we eat, but we cannot use the material unless we are sometimes at rest, and by quiescence of brain and muscle give a chance for worn-out cells to be removed and new material put in their place. It is when we lay our bodies down in the beautiful repose of slumber that this process can go on with most perfect results. Then, when all the forces can be concentrated on the process of nutrition, will nutrition be most perfect. When we awake refreshed after a night of sound sleep we are really fed. It is quite doubtful if, in a normal condition, we would want food until we had been at work some time and by destroying tissue have created a demand for more new material.

If we were only half as anxious that food should be assimilated—that is, made over into ourselves—as we are that it should be put into the stomach, we would be very careful to secure for ourselves a due amount of good sleep. And what is a due amount? That depends. I once heard of a servant girl whose mistress complained of her because she did not get up early in the morning, and the girl's excuse was, "But, ma'am, I can't get up early because I sleep so slow."

It seems a ridiculous statement, and yet there is a germ of truth in it. In some people the vital processes go on with such rapidity that the old, worn-out material will be eliminated and the new material built into the body in a comparatively short time. Seven hours of good sleep, perhaps, make them feel strong and rested and able to start on a new day's work with courage and ease. In others the vital processes are hindered or work feebly and slowly, and eight or nine hours of sleep scarcely suffice to complete the work of restoration. What is the obvious inference? Simply that each one shall judge for himself; but each should be wise enough not to confuse sleeplessness with having had sufficient sleep.

Very frequently the loss of sleep makes it difficult or impossible to sleep, and not until the excited condition of nerves can be calmed, can refreshing slumber be obtained. Young women who attempt to be in school and in society at the same time often bring themselves into the condition of insomnia or sleeplessness, and foolishly fancy that because they do not sleep they do not need it.

It is not at all difficult to understand that if you are constantly taking money out of the bank, you must also be constantly putting money in, or some day you will be told that your account is already overdrawn and your draft will not be honored. One can overdraw for a time, and right here is the danger with young people. They fancy, because they are not at once told that they are overdrawing, that their bank account is unlimited, and then, when it is too late, they find themselves on the verge, if not clear over the verge, of bankruptcy.

How shall you know whether you sleep enough? If you will make it a rule to go to bed by ten o'clock every night, and go to sleep at once, and sleep soundly and waken with a clear head and a rested feeling, you may infer that you have slept enough. If you are still tired or dull, something is wrong. You may have been in bed long enough, but your room may not have been ventilated, and so you may be poisoned by breathing over and over again the emanations from your own body. Or for some reason the process of digestion and assimilation may not have been carried on, and poisons have been created instead of being eliminated.

If you waken unrefreshed, I should want to inquire into your habits of life. Was there opportunity for fresh air to enter your room? Was there in it no uncovered vessel, no old shoes in the closet, no soiled underclothing, nothing that could contaminate the atmosphere? Did you eat a hearty supper late in the evening? Is your system oppressed with a superabundance of sweets? Are you living on simple, wholesome food, or eating irregularly of all sorts of trash? There may be many causes, you see, for your "tired feeling" in the morning, and instead of taking some "Sarsaparilla," or other drug, I should try to find out the cause and remove it.

Many people are afraid of night air, and scrupulously shut it out of their sleeping-rooms, and yet, what kind of air can you get at night but night air? And is it not better to have pure night air from out of doors than the impure night air of a close room? I once went with two ladies to ascend the Rigi in Switzerland, in order to see the sun rise. One of these was a Polish countess, who took with her a little black-and-tan terrier. The hotel at the Rigi Staeffel was crowded, and we thought ourselves very fortunate to secure a room with three beds. The Countess disposed herself in one bed with her little dog, and I took one bed, saying to my friend, "You'll please open the window before you go to bed?" "O certainly," she replied.

The little Countess sprang up in evident alarm. "Open the window!" she cried; "why, we'd all take our death of cold! I beg of you don't do it. I could not sleep a wink if the window were open."

My friend spoke reassuringly to her, and she at length grew quiet, when my friend surreptitiously raised a window and we went to sleep. The next morning the Countess asked, with a strange air of incredulity, "Were you in earnest when you spoke about opening the window? Why, I never heard of such a thing in my life. I know I should have been ill if you had persisted in having the window open."

My friend and I exchanged glances silently. We knew she was not ill and she had slept with the window open, but doubtless she would have been ill had she known it was open, for she had a wonderful imagination. When we were called at three o'clock to get up and go to the top of the mountain to see the sun rise, she turned herself luxuriously in her bed and said she could imagine it. She had taken this journey and "climbed the mountain" (that is, was carried up in a chair, with her dog in her lap), to see the famous sunrise on the Rigi, and then remained in bed and imagined it! Her imagination seemed entirely satisfactory, and so we did not quarrel with her.

Sleep is the most positive beautifier, the best cosmetic. The term "beauty sleep" is no misnomer. Sleep freshens the complexion,

What a Young Woman Ought to Know

smoothes out wrinkles, clears out the brain, strengthens the muscles, puts light into the eyes and color into the cheek.

CHAPTER V.

BREATHING.

The first thing you did when you came into this world was to inspire, that is, to breathe in. The last thing you will do will be to expire, that is, to breathe out. And between your first inspiration and your last expiration there will have been the process of respiration, that is, breathing in and out at an average rate of twenty times a minute. Twenty times a minute means twelve hundred times an hour, or nearly thirty thousand times a day, or over ten million times a year. If you should live to be fifty years old, you will have breathed in and out over five hundred million times. We eat three times a day, twenty-one times a week, over a thousand times a year, fifty thousand times in fifty years, but we breathe over five hundred million times in fifty years.

We realize the importance of eating, but we can live days without food. On the other hand, we cannot live many seconds entirely without air. We must infer from all this that breathing is more important than eating. How can it be? From our food our body is rebuilt. What life-process is accomplished by breathing?

To understand this, we must learn what processes are going on in the body, by means of which food is converted into tissue, into heat and energy. These processes we find are chemical, and may be likened to the combustion of wood or coal in the furnace. We know that fire must have air in order to burn. Burning is the process of oxidation or combustion of oxygen with the atoms of fuel and the formation of a new substance thereby. Coal, we are told, consists of carbon and nitrogen, both of which readily combine with oxygen, and in the process of uniting heat is liberated, and waste compounds thus formed pass off through the smokestack or chimney. We may not understand this scientifically, but we know that if we want the fire to burn well we must give it draft or air.

Our bodies are living engines, and use food and air instead of coal and air. Food in the body without air is like the coal in an engine without air; and air is useful only because it brings oxygen to unite chemically with the food. This process is going on all over the body. Each little microscopical cell is a furnace in which oxidation is taking place; and not only is energy liberated, but reconstructive processes are going on, new tissues are being formed, and old tissues removed.

But how can the oxygen get to the cells in all parts of the body? We can readily see how it gets to the air-cells of the lungs, but it would do little good if it stopped there. It must be carried in some way to all the minutest cells of all the tissues. This is done through the breathing. The blood goes to the lungs, and there it gives out the waste material it has collected in its journey through the body and takes up oxygen. The blood goes to the lungs dark in color from its load of waste. It is changed to a bright red by taking up oxygen. Each red blood-corpuscle takes a load of oxygen, carries it to its destination, and gives it to some tissue to be used up in the chemical process of oxidation, upon which depends our life and energy. During the hours of rest the tissues are busy in this process, and during exercise the energy stored up in the tissue-cells is liberated and waste created. So we see that the process is a continual round of taking food and air, using them in rebuilding tissue, then using up the tissue by exercise and casting out the waste products. And now we can begin to understand that we live in proportion as we breathe. Dr. Holbrook says: "The activity of the child is in close relation to the strength of its lungs; so, too, is the calmness, dignity and power of a man in proportion to the depth and tranquility of his respiration. If the lungs are strong and active, there is courage and boldness; if feeble, there is cowardice and debility. To be out of spirits is to be out of breath. To be animated and joyous is to be full of breath." "Breathing," writes Dr. von der Deeken, "is an actual vivifying act, and the need of breath as felt is a real life-hunger and a proof that without the continual charging of the blood-column with the proper force, all the other vital organs would soon stagnate and cease action altogether."

Now I wonder how many young women really know how to breathe. "Why," you say, "we have always breathed!" And I reply, "So you have, to some extent; but do you really breathe, or do you just let a little current of air flow gently through a part of your lungs, not reaching the minute air-cells at all, or have you crippled a large part of your lung-power by the restrictions of tight clothing?" Now you shrug your shoulders and say, with a little irritation, perhaps, "O, now she is going to scold about corsets and tight-lacing, and I do not wear my clothes tight." But I am not now going to talk of lacing; I am going to talk about singing, and speaking, and real living. The highest class of living creatures are those that have most power to breathe. The cold-blooded animals breathe little, and are slow-moving creatures with deficient sensation and small powers of action. Man has large lung-capacity and should be full of life and power, and will be, if he understands himself. One benefit of exercise is the added impulse given to the heart and lungs, calling for more breath, and bringing more blood to the lungs to receive the added supply of oxygen.

If we were wise we would practise the art of deep, voluntary breathing, as a daily form of gymnastics. What would it do for us? Wonderful things, if we may believe the doctors. Even in the old Greek and Roman times the doctors recommended deep breathing, the voluntary holding of air in the lungs, believing that this exercise cleansed the system of impurities and gave strength. And all our scientific discoverers have proven that they were right, and modern doctors have only learned more of the process and added to the wisdom of the ancients. Professor Lehwess says that he uses deep breathing not only as a health remedy but as a cure for muscular convulsions, especially chronic spasms; and he says that he bases his method for the cure of stuttering mainly upon respiratory and vocal exercises, "whereby," he says, "we work on enervated muscles, and make their function bring them into permanent activity and make them obedient to our will." Thus not only will the respiratory system be enlarged and quickened, and the lungs strengthened, but the blood circulation is promoted and those injurious influences overcome which often take away the stutterer's courage for speaking.

Dr. Niemeyer, of Leipzig, urges breathing in these words: "Prize air; use good, pure air; breathe fresh air in your room by night and day." Dr. Bicking says that respiratory gymnastics are the only effectual remedy for pulmonary affection, especially for consumption. The

Marquise Ciccolina claims that by the teaching of breathing gymnastics she has cured people of a tendency to take cold easily; she has benefited cases of lung and heart trouble, and she has cured nervous asthma even in cases that have lasted from childhood to maturity. Dr. Kitchen asserts that if the various structures of the body, including the lungs, are in a sufficiently healthy state, consumption cannot find a soil in which to commence its ravages, or, if already commenced, can be cured by attention to the general health, by pure air and deep breathing.

All this proves that the breathing is of great importance—of just as much importance to women as to men. It used to be thought that women breathe naturally with the upper part of the chest and men with the abdominal muscles, but we have now learned that in the breathing of both men and women the diaphragm should be used and the lower part of the chest expanded. The breathing should neither be thoracic—that is, with the upper part of the chest—nor abdominal. It should be diaphragmatic; that is, with the expansion of the sides of the lower part of the chest, thus filling every air-cell and bringing the life-giving oxygen to the blood. The importance of the diaphragm as the breathing muscle cannot be overestimated. A diaphragm, you know, is a partition across a cylinder; the diaphragm is a muscular partition across the cylinder of the body, dividing the lungs from the abdomen. In breathing, the diaphragm becomes tense, and in becoming tense becomes also flattened, just as an umbrella does by being opened. In fact the opening and shutting of an umbrella gives a very good idea of the motion of the diaphragm in breathing. We can realize, then, how much larger around the body will be when the lungs are fully inflated than it is when we breathe the air out and the lungs are empty. A few minutes spent each day in exercising in diaphragmatic breathing would be of great advantage in increasing beauty of form, in giving strength and power to the voice, in improving the complexion and adding to the health, and therefore to the happiness. In taking these exercises, one should either stand erect or lie flat upon the back and draw the air in through the nose, keeping the mouth closed. Draw in gently, allowing the chest to expand at the sides, hold the air for a little time, and then breathe out slowly.

These exercises performed in a room that is well ventilated, or, better still, in the pure air of outdoors, will do much toward driving away headaches, clearing the brain, giving better judgment, stronger will, and a clearer, happier, brighter disposition.

CHAPTER VI.

HINDRANCES TO BREATHING.

This little conversation will be on the hindrances to deep breathing, for if we make up our minds that it is so important to breathe deeply we shall be very anxious to know how to avoid the hindrances to deep breathing. First, let me speak of attitude. If you study physiology and note the arrangement of the internal organs, you will very easily see that when the body is compressed in a sitting attitude there must be a hindrance to full and deep breathing. The girl who is running the typewriter or the sewing-machine, or the girl who is working as bookkeeper or stenographer, or the girl at her studies, is sitting so that it will not be possible to breathe deeply, for the lungs are encroached upon by the crowding together of the other *viscera* (which means the vital organs) and the action of the breathing muscles is impeded by compression. As you will readily observe, there can be no lifting of the chest in this compressed attitude, no complete flattening of the diaphragm, no full inflation of the minute air-cells; therefore, as we have learned, the blood is not thoroughly purified, and actual poisons created by the vital processes accumulate in the brain and tissues until you feel overpoweringly weary and stupid. You cannot think, because you cannot fully breathe.

You have often found, when sewing, that the machine would get, as you say, bewitched. It wouldn't feed, the thread would break or the needle would snap, and the whole work go wrong. Put the machine away, take a rest, and the next day, without doing anything at all to the machine, you find that it runs perfectly. The trouble was with yourself. It is so with the girl who is running the typewriter. She finds that it makes mistakes in spelling, things go wrong altogether. It "acts up," as she would say. So with the girl who is bookkeeper. The figures will not add themselves up right. Now if, under these circumstances, the girl would get up, go to the door, take a few deep breaths and expand the lungs fully, she would relieve the internal congestion consequent upon the cramped position, the brain would be freed from the accumulated poison, and as a consequence the troublesome problems would soon be solved, the typewriter would spell correctly, the figures would add themselves up accurately, and life would become brighter at once. Five minutes spent each hour in deep breathing of pure air would add both to the quality and quantity of work done, and so be a saving of time. This certainly is of great value to you in your work in the world.

After working-hours are over, the girl should make a special effort to sit erect for other reasons than that of breathing, though that is reason enough.

But wrong sitting-postures are not the only attitudes that interfere with deep breathing. Very often the position in standing is also objectionable. When one stands with the weight resting on the heels the body is thrown out of balance, and as a consequence the shoulders are not on a vertical line with the hips. In this attitude it is impossible to manifest fullness of life, because the lungs are not fully inflated with air at each breath. We live, enjoy, accomplish only in proportion to our breathing ability. As one writer says, "The deep thinker, the orator, the fine singer, must of necessity be a good breather."

The most serious hindrance to deep breathing is found in the restrictions of the clothing. I do not say of the corsets, because tight bands or waists can also compress the body and make full breathing impossible. Of course you say your dresses are loose, and you run your hand up under your waist to prove it to me. I will not argue the question with you, but I will ask you to argue it with yourself.

If breathing is the measure of your living and doing, then if, in the least degree, you limit by your dress your breathing, the dress is too tight. "Well," you ask "how shall I know if I am hindering my breathing? My dress feels comfortable. It seems to me that I breathe. Is there any way that I can prove whether my dress is tight or not?"

It is true that one becomes accustomed to uncomfortable things and scarcely realizes that they ever were uncomfortable. The dress may seem a little tight when you first put it on, then it begins to grow comfortable, and after a while it feels loose, and you say it certainly is loose. I will give a simple rule by which you may know whether your clothing is loose enough or not. Unfasten every article of clothing; dress, corset, skirt-bands, everything. Now breathe in slowly until every air-cell is full. It may take some practice to do this, but persevere until you find the chest elevated and filled to its utmost extent. It should swell out at the sides along the line of the insertion of the diaphragm. There should be no heaving of the chest. Now, with the lungs so completely filled with air, bring your dress waist together without pulling a particle. Will it fasten without pressing out a bit of air from the lungs? If so, it is loose enough. If, however, you have to pull it together, even to the tiniest extent, you have pressed out some of the air. The minute air-cells that have thus been emptied cannot be again filled while the dress is fastened. Therefore you are defrauded of your rightful amount of air, and because part of the air is pressed out, the lungs take less space and the dress seems looser. You can understand how that would be.

The trouble is that our dresses are usually fitted over empty lungs. The dressmaker pulls the dress together, squeezes the air out of the lungs, and fastens the dress. Now you can readily understand that it will be impossible to fill those air-cells so long as the dress is worn, and yet it may not seem uncomfortable, because we become accustomed to it. Nature has made us so that we can accustom ourselves to many things that are not absolutely healthful, but this should not make us willing to live unhealthfully when it is possible to avoid it.

CHAPTER VII.

ADDED INJURIES FROM TIGHT CLOTHING.

We have talked of the effect of tight clothing upon the breathing power. Let us see what other injuries arise from wearing the dress too tight. In the first place, the action of the heart is impeded. The heart is a hollow muscle which must be continually filled with blood and emptied again many times a minute from the moment of birth till the moment of death. You have been lying down for an hour; let me count your pulse. Now sit up for a few moments. I find, now, that it beats faster. Now stand up, and it beats still faster. You see, it increases continually as you get into the erect position. Now walk quickly across the floor and you will see how much it has increased again in rapidity.

You will realize how much the dress interferes with the action of the heart better from an illustration. Professor Sargent made an experiment with a number of girls. One day they were dressed in perfectly loose clothing. He counted the pulse of each. It beat on the average of eighty-four times in a minute. He had them run five hundred and forty yards in the space of two and a half minutes. The pulse was again counted. It had increased to one hundred and fifty-six beats in a minute. This illustrates the effect of exercise even in loose clothing. The next day at the same time, dressed with a corset which reduced the waist to twenty-four inches, they ran the same distance in the same length of time, and then he found that the pulse had run up to one hundred and sixty-eight beats in a minute, showing how much harder it was for the heart to do its work when restricted by tight clothing. No acrobat would attempt to perform feats of strength or of agility if restricted even so much as by a belt.

The Russian Government has issued an edict that the soldiers must wear their pantaloons held up by suspenders, for it has been demonstrated that when they wear them supported by a belt around the waist they are not able to do a fair amount of work. The Austrian Government has also decreed that the pantaloons of soldiers are not to be suspended by belts because of the increase of kidney difficulty caused thereby.

We will understand why kidney difficulty is caused by tight clothing when we study the location of the kidneys and how they are affected by compression of the ribs. Most people think the kidneys lie low down in the back, but in reality they lie up under the short ribs, and the pressure of tight clothing brings the ribs to bear directly upon the kidneys, injuring them in such a way as often to cause disease.

The heart and lungs are protected by a bony framework called the thorax, but below the thorax there is no protection for the internal organs except that of the muscles, therefore the corset or tight clothing can do most damage to the vital organs below the diaphragm. The largest of these is the liver. It should lie close up under the diaphragm, from which it is suspended. Under the influence of tight clothing it is often pressed over on the right side, sometimes extending over the whole front of the body, or even as low down as the navel. It is rutted by the pressure of the ribs. The corset liver is well known in the dissecting-room. Sometimes, where corsets are not worn and tight skirts are worn, supported by the hips, the liver has almost been cut in two, the pieces being only held together by a sufficient band of tissue to keep them from dying.

When Hiram Powers, the great sculptor, was in this country, he once attended an elegant party, and was observed watching very intently a beautifully dressed, fashionable woman. A friend, noticing his interest, said to him, "What an elegant figure she has, hasn't she?"

"Well," said Powers, "I was wondering where she put her liver."

You see, Powers had studied the human body, and when he saw such an outline as the figure of a fashionable woman, he knew that some internal organ must be displaced in order to create that tapering waist, and his anxiety was for the internal organs. As an artist he did not admire the tapering waist, as is shown by the beautiful marble statue which he made. No artist would perpetuate in marble the figure of the fashionable woman.

Not only is the liver thus displaced, but the stomach is often pressed out of its original position, which should be also close up under the diaphragm, towards the left side. By the pressure of clothing it is sometimes pushed down until it lies in the abdominal cavity, even as low down as the navel. This is the statement of Dr. J.H. Kellogg, who, in his sanitarium at Battle Creek, examines hundreds, or even thousands of women in a year, and asserts that it is almost impossible to find a woman whose stomach is where it belongs. This is a serious matter, because no organ can do its work properly when it is out of its rightful position. We understand this in any machinery except that of the human body. We would not meddle with a man-made machine because that would hinder its perfect working, but we do not hesitate to interfere with the body, forgetful that it, too, is a machine, divinely created, and with powers most fateful to us for weal or woe.

But the harm is not all done by the displacement of the organs mentioned. The bowels suffer, and we can best understand what is done to them when we understand how they are placed in the abdominal cavity.

Let me take the ruffle you are making. The mesentery is a delicate, narrow membrane about twenty feet long. We will compare it to the ruffle. Folded in it at one edge are the small intestines, just as I can run this bodkin into the hem of this ruffle. The other edge of the mesentery is gathered up as you have gathered the ruffle. It is gathered into a space of about six inches in length, and is fastened up and down the spine in the region of the small of the back. You can see, if I gather up twenty feet of this ruffle into a space of six inches, how the mesentery, with the intestines folded in the free edge, are held in the abdominal cavity. They are held loosely, and at the same time so that the intestines cannot be tied in knots or loops upon each other. In this way the ruffle flares out into the abdominal cavity. The intestines should stay in their place close up under the liver and stomach, but if pressure is brought to bear around the body at this point, the bowels begin to sag into the abdominal cavity. The abdominal walls lose their tonicity because they are so compressed that they cannot have a perfect circulation, the bowels sink down still further into the pelvis, and pull upon their attachment in the small of the back, creating backache. The stomach sags down into the cavity; the liver sinks, and all the organs pull upon their attachments; so it is no wonder that women have backaches and headaches, and their eyes feel bad, and they are unable to stand or walk. We don't want small rooms in our dwelling-houses, we don't like it if we haven't sufficient space for our furniture; but in this bodily house in which we dwell we are quite willing to constrict the rooms in which the vital organs or furniture are placed, until everything is huddled together in the closest pressure, so that the organs are unable to do their work. It wouldn't matter in our parlors if the chairs and tables were huddled close together, for they are not constantly changing in size, but it does matter in a room where machines must have space to work and such space is not permitted them; and we cannot expect good work where we crowd machinery so that it does not have adequate room.

The influence of tight clothing upon the pelvic organs is to displace them and create a great many difficulties which we know as "Female Diseases." But these, in my opinion, are not the most important things. The important things are the displacement of the vital organs of the body—those organs without which we cannot live, and those organs the perfect working of which is necessary both to our health and our happiness. If we are wise we will be exceedingly anxious that every vital organ shall be allowed to hold its own position, to do its own work, with plenty of room.

The impeding of the heart-action by tight clothing is not in itself the most serious effect of this restriction. The serious trouble is in the disturbance of the circulation. Upon a perfect circulation depends perfect nutrition. The blood must go in sufficient quantity to every organ in order that it may be fully nourished. When the waist is compressed the organs do not receive their full amount of blood. It is retained, and therefore the organs are congested. The feet are cold because the blood does not reach them in sufficient quantity, and the brain, it may be, is hot, because the blood is not taken from the head with enough rapidity and furnished to the other organs. So we find that tight clothing interferes with the integrity and health of every organ in the body, and consequently with our happiness and with our usefulness.

The reason we admire the tapering waist is because we have been wrongly educated. We have acquired wrong ideas of beauty. We have accepted the ideals of the fashion-plate rather than those of the Creator. We find that some form of physical deformity maintains in almost every country. The Chinese deform the feet, and we think this is barbarous, but it is really not as serious as the deforming of the vital parts of the body. The Flathead Indian is deformed in babyhood by being compressed between boards until the head changes its shape. Among some savage nations the leg is bandaged for a few inches above the ankle and for a few inches below the knee and the central part is allowed to expand as it will, and this deformity to them constitutes beauty. Among other nations, holes are made in the ears and pieces of wood are inserted. The size of these pieces is gradually increased until the lobe of the ear will hang down upon the shoulder and a piece of wood as large as a man's arm be worn in the ears. All of these things seem to us most horrible; yet, after all, they are not as much an insult to the Divine Architect of the body as the deformity practised by civilized and so-called Christian people, who by restriction of the waist interfere with the vital organs and prevent the body from being perfect in its development, or perfect in its action. The activity of the body is an evidence of its life, and if it is so tied up that it cannot be active, it certainly is not in the fullest condition of life.

CHAPTER VIII.

EXERCISE.

You said to me, my daughter, that you wanted to join the class in Physical Culture. I asked you why, and you said because you thought you needed to build up in certain parts of the body. You were defective in muscular development; you needed also to acquire grace, you thought. And I said, "Is muscular development the primary object of physical education?" You seemed to think that it is. Now I want to talk to you a little along that line, and to demonstrate to you, if I can, that physical education is not primarily for the building up of big muscle, or for the gaining of power to do great feats of bodily strength or skill. The object of physical education is to develop a quickly responsive, flexible instrument for the soul to use, for that is what the body is. Physical culture, rightly conducted, aims to secure the highest condition of the body through the exercises that are required by the laws of the body. Law, physical law, governs the body, and exercise should be according to this law. The first object of exercise is to make a vital supply for the whole body. This is first secured by proper attitude. If we stand or sit properly we gain a proper position of the vital organs, and then they will do their work well, and the result will be more perfect nutrition.

The use of certain organs increases supply, and the use of others quickens waste; a balance should be maintained between the two. We must nourish the life-sustaining organs before using the organs which use up brain-supply, therefore we want to be sure that we are working according to these laws. A great many people have an idea that physical culture means building up big muscle. They measure the muscles of the arm and of the leg, and judge by their increase in size of the value of the exercise. This is not a correct measurement. Individuals may weigh themselves down by development of muscles until they have not sufficient internal vital force to carry so much weight. If we could only balance between the organs which supply nutriment and the organs which use it up, we would keep in perfect health.

We want to learn how to secure a maximum of results with a minimum of force. That is, we want the body to be quickly responsive, to be flexible, to be so that we can use it for the things we want to do without wasting strength, and yet without being weighed down by a superabundance of muscular tissue.

The first desideratum in taking exercise is to have every organ of the body free, therefore a gymnastic dress is a necessity. Then we should have the exercise conducted by some one who understands the peculiarities of each individual and knows just what exercises are suited for her in her special physical condition. They should also be directed by one who understands perfectly that the girl with an anæmic brain, that is, with a brain having too little blood, cannot be conducted on the same plan as the exercise of the girl who has a superabundance of blood in the brain.

The best exercise is that which employs the mind pleasantly. A good deal of exercise may be obtained in housework, and, if conducted with pleasure in the work, may be of great physical advantage. Not long ago I listened to a very charming talk by a lady whose dress betokened her a woman of society. She wore white kid gloves, a dainty flower bonnet, and in herself appeared an exponent of leisure and happiness. Her address was entitled "The Home Gymnasium," and I supposed that it would consist of descriptions of machinery that could be put up in one's own dwelling for gymnastic purposes, but I soon found that her home gymnasium meant household duties. She said one could scrub the table and obtain the best exercise for arms and chest, and at the same time produce an article or piece of furniture which would be a delight to the eye in its whiteness and brightness. She said that in scrubbing the floor one obtained very much the same movement that would be given in the gymnasium, while at the same time the exercise would conduce not only to the personal advantage but to the happiness of the family. She spoke of sweeping, and dusting, and bed-making, and expressed herself as competent to do all these kinds of work, in fact, as doing them. And she said she never felt more of a lady than when scrubbing her kitchen floor, and she was not ashamed to be seen by her friends at this work. If any one rang the door-bell, she said she would simply put on a clean apron and go to the door, and remark without hesitation that she was just scrubbing her kitchen floor, but she was glad to see her friends.

This sort of a home gymnasium is at the command of nearly every girl, and if she can bring herself to feel an interest in this home gymnastic exercise, she may find it conducive not only to her own physical well-being, but to the comfort and happiness of all about her.

The question is often asked whether bicycle-riding is injurious for girls, and I would say that in my opinion it depends largely upon the girl. Has she good common sense? Of course I am speaking of the girl who is in a normal condition of health. A girl of extreme delicacy, or who is subject to some functional difficulty, or the victim of some organic disease, might not find it advantageous to ride. A physician should, in these cases, be consulted. But for the ordinary girl, the girl of fairly good health, if she will learn how to sit properly upon her saddle, will have the good sense to ride with judgment, it seems to me that the exercise must be productive of great good.

My own experience is somewhat limited. I made some discoveries in my attempts to ride. In the first place, I learned that it was important to know how to sit. In reading a book on "Physical Culture and Hygiene for Women," by Dr. Anna Galbraith, I found this sentence: "Sit upon the gluteal muscles, and not upon the perineum." This was a revelation to me. I found that I had been doing the thing which was not proper, and bearing the weight almost entirely upon the perineum had caused constant rectal irritation. The gluteal muscles, closely held together, form a firm support for the body without injuring any of the vital organs. I found that by distributing the weight—a little upon the handle-bars, and some upon the feet—I was able to sit with less weight and heaviness upon the saddle. I found, too, that it was quite important to have the saddle high enough, so that the legs might be fully extended at each stroke, and with these precautions I found the wheel a source both of enjoyment and of strength.

The harm done by the wheel I believe in most instances to be due to an ill-adapted saddle or a lack of good judgment in the amount of exercise taken. It is such a fascinating exercise, one seems to be flying and scarcely realizes how much of nerve-force is being expended. If the girl learning to ride will be prudent, gauging the amount of exercise by her amount of strength; if she will gradually acquire the needed strength before attempting long wheeling trips; if she will be judicious and not ride, perhaps, during the first two or three days of menstruation, there seems to be no reason why the ordinary girl should not be entirely benefited by this most delightful form of exercise. It is not as objectionable, to any degree, as the exercise of dancing. Dancing is a most fascinating amusement, and if it only could be conducted under proper circumstances it would be very delightful. In itself it is not so objectionable as in its concomitants; the late hours, the improper dressing, the hearty suppers in the middle of the night, the promiscuous association and the undue familiarity of the attitude of the round dance are what make dancing objectionable. If dancing could be conducted out of doors, in the daylight, with intimate friends, without the round dances, only those forms of dancing which may be likened to gymnastics, as the contra-dance, the cotillion, the objections to dancing would be largely removed, but I am of the opinion that a large share of the fascination of dancing would go at the same time.

Skating is a delightful, invigorating form of exercise, if conducted with judgment. One objection to it is that the girl will skate until wearied, and then, in that exhausted condition, perhaps ride home, or take a long, tiresome walk from the pond to her residence, all of which is sapping her unduly and annulling the value of the skating as an exercise.

Lawn-tennis is delightful and beneficial, provided it is undertaken with due judgment and the girl is properly dressed. In fact, the subject of dress is so closely associated with that of exercise that they can never be considered separately. Even the moderate exercise of walking, conducted in the dress of the fashionable woman, is in itself an element of danger, whereas more violent exercise in a loose dress becomes a means of increased strength and vigor.

I am often asked if girls should be allowed to run up and down stairs. I see no reason why girls should not go up and down stairs just as freely as boys, if they are properly dressed; but going up and down stairs in tight clothing is certainly very injurious.

CHAPTER IX.

BATHING.

You and your girl friends take much pains with your personal adornment. You spend time in curling your hair and in putting on ribbons and laces, but I sometimes think you do not pay as much attention to personal cleanliness as you ought. It would seem as if some of you thought that powder would cover a defect in cleanliness and perfumery would conceal the odors of the person; but indeed it seems to me that the stylish make-up of your dress or the curl of your hair is of very little importance compared with the care of your health.

You each desire to have a beautiful complexion. I used to be told in my childhood that beauty was only skin-deep, but I have learned better. I know that even the beauty of the complexion depends upon the integrity of the nutritive organs as well as upon the care and attention given to matters of personal cleanliness.

I read the other day of a discussion between two young men concerning the cleanliness of girls of their acquaintance. One young man noticed that although one of the girls wore a very pretty dress-gown, she had forgotten to clean her finger-nails. The other remarked that many things in regard to a girl's personal cleanliness could be learned by riding behind her on a tandem. The two then commented favorably upon the girl whose nails were pink, whose ears and neck were clean, her teeth white and dazzling, and her hair well brushed. I might say, in passing, that this hair-brushing time at night may be well employed in reviewing the experiences of the day in order to learn the lessons they teach, and thereby to avoid to-morrow the mistakes of to-day.

These same young men also said that the complexions of some girls suggested the idea of too little fresh air and too much candy. This, they agreed, it was impossible to hide with powder. So we see that the care of the skin is quite important if one would have the respect and the admiration of her associates.

The skin is a very beautiful, complex and delicate covering of the body. It consists of six layers, and contains arteries, capillaries, lymphatics, nerves, sweat glands, sebaceous glands, pigment, etc. So you see that the care of the skin involves much. One writer has said, "At the skin man ends and the outlying universe begins."

The skin, filled with nerves, is continually reporting to the brain concerning what is the condition of all parts of the body. The condition of the skin reflects the condition of the digestive organs. Many girls are trying to cure pimples on the face by the use of salves and lotions, when in all probability all that they would need to do to gain a good complexion is to pay attention to diet, to quit eating between meals, and not to eat so much pastry, pickles or sweetmeats. Our athletes and pugilists are learning that they must take care of the skin if they would keep in good condition, and they are what in horses would be called well groomed. The skin is rubbed, cared for, kept active, because it is understood that it is an organ of sensation, of secretion, of excretion, of absorption, and of respiration. More solid matter is thrown out from the skin than from the lungs, in the proportion of eleven to seven. It is even more than the excretion from the bowels.

The skin is an organ of breathing. This seems strange to us, but it really does take up oxygen and give out carbonic acid, so upon the condition of the skin will depend very largely the condition of the general health. We can detect a constipated condition of the bowels through the color and odor of the skin.

Many girls feel that it is more delicate to neglect the care of the bowels than to attend to a daily evacuation, but if they would remember that it is just as indelicate to carry effete or dead matter about in the bowels as it would be to carry it upon the person in any other way, they would realize that it is only politeness and refinement to see that this part of their bodily housekeeping is duly attended to. If the bowels do not do their work the skin will be obliged to take extra labor upon itself; so, as we have said, by the odor of the skin we can detect the fact that the skin is doing the work that should be done by the bowels. When a person is sick the condition of the internal organs is shown in the complexion, and nothing more clearly indicates health than the condition of the skin.

If this is so important, how shall we care for the skin? First, by bathing. The tin bath-tub of the Englishman accompanies him in all his travels, and has penetrated even to the jungles of Africa. Bathing appliances are marks of civilization, and the bath-room is becoming a necessity. Where the bath-room does not exist it is easy to bathe thoroughly and completely. A wash-basin of water, with a sponge and towel, furnish all that is absolutely necessary. A most convenient bath is the portable thermal bath, an arrangement of rubber cloth that can be opened out to form a square enclosure in which the person sits, with the head in the free outside air, the body enveloped in steam generated by an alcohol lamp. This, followed by a quick sponge-bath of cool water, is a most efficient way of cleansing the skin; and this bath may be used in any room, no matter how beautifully furnished, without soiling the carpet or furniture in the least.

One great secret of healthful bathing is, when warm or hot water is used, to follow it by an immediate application of cold water, which leaves the skin in a tonic condition. In preparation for going out in cold weather, nothing is so efficient a protection from the cold as a foot-bath. Soak the feet for a few minutes in water as warm as is comfortable, then plunge them into cold water and remove immediately, or throw cold water over them, wipe them thoroughly dry, rub them with a little olive oil, draw on a pair of clean, warm hose, and the feet are not only warmed, but are protected against cold and will stay warm. These precautions will prevent one taking cold from the foot-bath. Care of the feet is a great necessity not only for health, for equalizing the circulation, but for the prevention of unpleasant odors.

As to time of bathing, I suppose that the body is at its highest point of vital power at about ten o'clock in the morning, but this is, for most people, the most inconvenient time for a bath. The circumstances of the individual are to be consulted, and also the effect of bathing. There are those who are made nervous by taking a bath, consequently they will not be benefited by taking one just before going to bed. In other cases the bath conduces to slumber. This depends very largely upon the amount of blood in the brain. A person with an anæmic brain will not be benefited by the bath at bedtime, but the person whose brain is overcharged with blood will find the evening bath quieting.

I would not advise everybody to take a daily bath. There are those who are benefited by it; there are others who might be injured by it. It is best to study personal peculiarities and to watch the effect of the bath. If, within a few hours, or the next day, there is great exhaustion, one might naturally conclude that the bath was not altogether beneficial. There are those in such delicate health that a cold bath at any time does not seem desirable; but constant attention will secure perfect cleanliness, as the arms and chest can be bathed one day, the abdomen and back another, the lower extremities still another day, and so the whole body be compassed twice or more in the space of a week.

In regard to the use of soap for bathing purposes, the finest, purest soaps should be used, and these alone. It is generally supposed that pure, white castile soap is the best. Various soaps are widely advertised, while some that claim to be of the very best are not always up to the requisite standard. Yet one can tell by a little experience what soap is of pure quality, and such soap can be applied even to the face without injury.

In washing the face the hand is probably the best instrument, with the thumb under the chin, the fingers turned toward the upper part of the face. The manipulation should be against the direction of forming wrinkles, wherever there is a tendency for wrinkles to appear. They can be held in check by the judicious manipulation of the fingers in the opposite direction. Wrinkles are created by obliterating the capillary circulation of the skin. The manipulation increases the circulation, and so tends to overcome wrinkles. The expression of the face may form wrinkles. I saw a girl the other day on a street-car who continually held her eyebrows elevated, forming longitudinal lines across her forehead, which had become as fixed in her youthful face as if she had been seventy years of age. This was a lack of care in the governing of the expression of the face, and also a lack in keeping up the capillary circulation.

The care of the hands may be considered also while discussing the question of bathing. The hands should be kept clean, the finger-nails particularly cared for, as much of the beauty of the hands depends upon the delicate appearance of the finger-nails. The manicure sets, which are at the disposal of almost every young woman of the present day, are a very great addition to toilet appurtenances. The curved scissors, the polisher, the blunt ivory instrument for pushing back the fold of skin from the root of the nail, all of these used but a few moments in the day will conduce to great beauty in the hands, even for those who are doing housework.

PART II.
NEED OF SPECIAL KNOWLEDGE; SOME FORMS OF AVOIDABLE DISEASE, THEIR REMEDY AND PREVENTION.

CHAPTER X.

CREATIVE POWER.

It is a wonderful thought that God shares His divine endowments with man; that He, being our Father, hath bestowed upon us the power to manifest His characteristics. We are proud of these Godlike powers. We talk of our Godlike reason, and it is divine. We know that God reasons. We have evidence of it in the material world about us, and when we use our reason we are "thinking God's thoughts after Him."

God has the marvelous power of imagination, using that word in its noblest sense. He has the power to conceive something in thought before it actually exists. He must have seen all the glories of the material universe, worlds upon worlds circling through space, moon and stars, the beauty of forest and stream, of tinted flower and iridescent insect wing before they were brought into being, and He had the power to create them. Man has this wonderful gift of imagination. The inventor sees the machine in his thought before he attempts to build it. The poet has the germ of his poem in mind, even the rhythm and rhyme, before he puts it on paper. To the imagination of the artist the canvas glows with color before his brush has touched it. The sculptor, looking at the rough block of marble, sees within it the imprisoned shape of beauty which his genius shall liberate to delight the world. The musician hears, singing through his brain, the marvelous harmonies which, put upon paper, shall entrance all hearers. Certainly this glorious gift of imagination is Godlike. But it would be useless if it were not accompanied by creative power. The inventor must be able to create as well as to imagine the engine. The poet, the musician, the artist fails of deserving the name if he cannot embody his thought in a form that others may recognize. He must not only imagine, but create. In some degree every intelligent human being has these powers. The housewife imagines her dinner before she prepares it, and a well-cooked dinner, placed upon a well-appointed table with care and taste, manifests something of the ability of the inventor and the artist. The same may be said of her who designs and creates an elegant costume, or arranges a room with taste and skill.

We appreciate the housewife's culinary creation; we admire the tasteful creation of the dressmaker; we wonder at the glorious creation of artist or musician; perhaps we even envy them. But food and clothing pass away and are forgotten. Even the grand symphony, the beautiful picture, the graceful statue, may pass into oblivion, and man forget that they ever existed.

But humanity is endowed with creative powers that are not transient. The brains builded by the individual are transmitted to his posterity from generation to generation.

God's greatest power is that of conferring life, sentient life. We might have imagined that that marvelous power he would have kept for Himself alone, but He has not done so. We have also the power to confer life. We can call into existence other human beings, and endow them with the record of our own lives, giving to them our form, our features, our measure of vitality, our tendencies, our habits; and these human beings whom we have thus called into life will never die. What diviner, more responsible gift could God have conferred upon us than this? What more worthy of our devout study? In this reverent attitude of mind let us study this gift of creative power, learning what we may of its scope and purpose and the material organs through which it works.

In your study of physiology in school you took up the organs of individual life. You studied the framework of the body, its machinery, its internal vital mechanism. You studied about digestion, nutrition, respiration, elimination, and in this you learned nothing of physical differences between individuals. All were considered as having the same organs, used in the same way. Girls have the same number of bones as boys, the same number of muscles, of vital organs. They sleep, breathe, eat, digest, grow, according to the same plan. So far there seems no reason why there should be any distinction of male and female. But as we come to study what is called special physiology we discover physical differences and reasons for their existence.

There are certain differences of form that are discernible at a glance. Men are usually larger than women. They have heavier bones and bigger muscles. They have broad shoulders and narrow hips, and have hair upon the face. Women have smooth faces, more rounded outlines, narrower shoulders and broader hips. In man the broadest part of the body is at the shoulders, in woman at the hips. This is significant of a great fact which will be manifest to you when you understand the functions of each sex. Although each has the same general plan of individual life, there are special functions which determine the trend of their lives. The man's broad shoulders are indicative that he is to bear the heavy burdens of life—struggles for material support—and woman's broad hips indicate that she is to bear the heavier burden of the race.

When we come fully to understand the deep significance of sex, we shall find in it a wonderful revelation of possibilities of development into a God-likeness that will stir our hearts to their very depths.

Humanity so weak, so lacking in appreciation of his possibilities, so groveling when he should soar, has been endowed with powers that give him control over the destiny of the race. We may well exclaim, with Young:

> "How poor, how rich, how abject, how august,
> How complicate, how wonderful is man!
> How passing wonder He who made him such!
> Who centred in his make such strange extremes!
> From diff'rent natures, marvelously mix'd!
> Connection exquisite of distant worlds!
> Distinguish'd link in being's endless chain!
> Midway from nothing to the Deity!"

CHAPTER XI.

BUILDING BRAINS.

When you were born you were, as all babies are, deaf, dumb, blind, and helpless, but immediately the external world began to act upon you. Then began the process of mind-building. You began to experience sensations of heat and cold, of hunger, of pain. The eyes began at once to recognize the light, the ears to become aware of sounds. After a time, objects were made clear to your sight and certain sounds were recognized. You learned your mother's face and voice, and, little by little, became acquainted with all the objects in the world of home. You began to use your limbs, and in this also you were at work building your mind. We do not sufficiently realize that every aimless movement of the baby has in reality a great purpose—that of creating brainpower sufficient to enable the baby to control itself in all its voluntary movements. We do not think that the fluttering hands and little kicking feet are really building brains, but this is so. And all of life's experiences have been building brain for you ever since.

Professor Elmer Gates tells us that only about ten per cent. of our brains are cultivated, that there is a vast field of brain possibilities lying undeveloped in each one of us, and that these possibilities are to be developed through cultivation of the senses. So while I have been talking to you of the care of your body, I have been advocating that which will in reality develop mind.

We have learned that certain areas of brain govern certain movements of body. For example, anatomists know not only where the general motor area is located, but they can indicate the very spot where any special motor-force is generated.

In the case of a mill girl who was subject to epilepsy and had pain in her right thumb at each attack, it was decided to remove the part of the brain which governed the motions of that thumb. This they could do because they knew just where that motor-center lies, and yet they were able to take out no more than that, for when the wound was healed she had full use of all of her hand except the thumb.

We may know that by exercising a certain organ we are building up a certain part of the brain. For example, the man who has cultivated his hearing until he can hear sounds inaudible to ordinary men, has made for himself more brain-cells in the hearing area. If he has cultivated his sight assiduously, he has created more visual cells. If his touch has been cultivated, his brain has received new touch sensation-cells. And Professor Gates asserts that his mental ability has been thereby increased. You will be interested in hearing of his experiments with animals and what he has learned therefrom.

He says he has demonstrated that it is possible to give to an animal or a human being more brains, and consequently a better use of the mental faculties. During twelve months, for five or six hours a day, he trained dogs to discriminate colors. He placed several hundred tin pans, painted different tints, in the yard with the dogs. At one time he put their food under pans of a certain tint. When they had learned to go at once to these pans for their food, he changed the color. Again he arranged it so that they would receive an electric shock if they touched pans of any color save the particular one. They soon learned to avoid all the pans except those of this tint. So, by many different methods, he trained them to recognize shades and tints until they could discriminate between seven shades of red and as many shades of green, and in many ways they manifested more mental ability than any untrained dog. While these dogs were being trained, another group of dogs were being deprived of the use of sight by being kept in a darkened room.

At the end of the year both groups of dogs were killed and their brains dissected. He found that the dogs kept in the darkness had less than the usual number of cells in the seeing areas, and the cells were smaller, while the dogs which had been trained to discriminate between tints and shades of color many times a day had a far greater number of larger and more complex brain-cells in the seeing areas than any dog of that age and species ever had before. "Therefore," says Professor Gates, "mind activity creates organic structure."

Prof. Gates discovered other things of equal importance. He carried his observations to successive generations, and found that the fifth generation was born with a far greater number of brain-cells than could be found in animals not descended from trained ancestors.

This is not only interesting, but of value. You will remember, in our talk concerning your value, we spoke of your value to the race, and learned that in cultivating yourself in any direction you were adding to the welfare of future generations. That was only a general statement, and now you can see how it can be. You see that if you can make more brains for yourself you are also making more brains for your posterity. Or if you fail to make brains for yourself, posterity will in like degree be defrauded.

Many people have the idea that we are obliged to be satisfied with our dower of mental ability, and so are excusable for failing to reach as high a level as some others. If we really believed that we could create brains we would not sit down and sigh over small mental capacity, but go to work at once in building minds for ourselves.

And first, we must learn to control our thoughts and make them go where we send them. In too many cases thoughts wander here and there, with no power governing and guiding them.

When we are sauntering in the wood we sometimes come upon pathways, and we know at once that many, many footsteps of men or animals have been needed to make the paths. If those who walked here had wandered each in his own way, no path would have been made. One pair of feet going often over the same ground will make a path. So the thoughts, traversing the same areas of brain, will make records on the brain-cells which we may call paths. Every time a thought follows the same line it creates a deeper impression, and makes it easier to go over the same territory again. In this way habits are formed. If the thoughts are good, the habits will be good; if evil, the habits will be bad.

It is not hard to understand how much easier it is to form a habit than to overcome it. The emotions, like the thoughts, create habits; but, more than this, they create actual physical conditions.

It was my pleasure and profit once to have a conversation with Professor Gates in his laboratory, and he showed me an instrument wherein he condenses the breath. He then subjects it to a chemical reagent, and by the precipitate formed he knows what was the mental condition of the individual, whether he were angry, sorrowful or remorseful. In five minutes after a fit of anger he finds the excretory organs beginning to throw out the poison which anger has created. Only five minutes suffice to create the poison, but half an hour is none too much to eliminate it.

Think what must be the bodily state of one who is constantly irritated or angry, who feels jealousy, hatred, or revenge. With body poisoned by these malevolent passions he cannot feel well, for his physical organs cannot do good work unless fed by pure blood. Professor Gates finds that the benevolent emotions create life-giving germs in the body; so, to love others is not only helpful to them, but it also gives us new life.

Anger, worry, hatred, jealousy, are suicidal emotions. We cannot for our own sakes afford to indulge in them, while from selfish reasons alone we should be incited to kindness, generosity, sympathy, and love.

CHAPTER XII.

YOU ARE MORE THAN BODY OR MIND.

We have talked of your body and your mind, but as yet not of yourself. You are not body; you are not mind; but you possess both. You are spirit, created by God, who is spirit; therefore you are His child. You may not have thought much of this fact, but that has not changed the fact. No failure to recognize God as your father changes His relationship to you. No conduct of yours can make you any less His child.

"Well," you may say, "if that is so, what does it matter, then, what I do? If disobedience or sin cannot make me less God's child, why should I be good and obedient?" Because, dear heart, your conduct changes your attitude towards Him. You might not know that I am your mother; you might know it and choose to disobey my wishes; yet in both cases I should still be your mother, and no more or less in one case than in the other. But you will have no difficulty in understanding that in one case you would be a loving, helpful, obedient daughter, a comfort and delight to me; in the other, a disobedient, willful, unloving daughter, a care and trouble.

We are God's children, each of us, dependent on His love and bounty for protection, food, friends, intellect, even life. Is it dignified and noble in us to ignore and disobey Him? Indeed the most worthy and dignified thing we can do is to recognize ourselves as God's children and be obedient. It is a wonderful glory to be a child of God. It means that we have Godlike powers. The children of human parents are like them in their capacities. Children of God must have capacities that are Godlike.

This is true even of the most ignorant or degraded. They have in themselves divine possibilities.

If you can get this thought fully engrafted into your consciousness, it seems to me you can never willfully do wrong, can never condescend to a mean or ignoble deed, because you recognize your divine inheritance, and feel compelled by it to live truly, nobly.

Being children of God puts on us certain obligations towards Him, but it also puts on God certain obligations towards us. "What!" you say; "God the Infinite under obligations to man, the finite? The Creator under obligations to the created?" Oh, yes.

We recognize the fact that human parents are under obligations to care for their children, to protect them, to educate them, to give them opportunities. Even such are the obligations of God towards His human children, and He fulfills them. All our earthly blessings are from His hand. Home, friends, shelter, food, are gifts of His love. He takes such minute care of us that if for one second of time He would forget us, we should be annihilated. He educates us. He does not send us away to a boarding-school where we hear from Him but seldom, but He has a home-school where He is both Father and Teacher, and His methods of instruction are divinely wise.

The injudicious love of earthly parents often induces them to do for their children things it would be far better to let the children do for themselves. I once knew a boy of seven years, as intelligent as the ordinary child, who had never been allowed to go down stairs alone in his life for fear he would fall. This unwise care of the parents had resulted in the child's being timid, fearful, and unable to care for himself. He would cry if he fell, and would lie still sobbing until some one came to pick him up and quiet him with caresses. At the same time I saw a boy of four who could run up and down stairs, go to the store alone to make purchases, and who, if he fell, would jump up quickly, saying, "O, that didn't hurt." Which child had been better protected—the one who had been cared for by an overindulgent parent, or the one who, by judicious stimulation to self-help, had learned to care for himself?

God teaches us how to help ourselves, and circumstances of life which we so often think hard and cruel are only the means by which we are being trained to be strong. The things we call failure, worriment, and hardship, are only the little tumbles by which we are learning to walk.

The heathen philosopher, Seneca, says: "God gives His best scholars the hardest lessons." We know how proud we would feel if our school-teacher would say, "This is a hard problem, but I believe you can solve it." We would be stimulated to work night and day to justify his confidence in our ability. But when a little trial comes in life we are quite apt to say, "God is so hard in His dealings with me. Why should He be so unkind?" instead of saying: "These hard things of life are a test of my scholarship, and are an evidence of my Teacher's confidence in my ability."

I would like you to get this thought fixed in your mind so firmly that you will feel sure that all circumstances of life are but lessons in God's great school, and, rightly used, will be the means of promoting you to higher grades.

No scholar wants to stay always in the primary department because it is easy there. He welcomes each promotion, although he knows it means harder lessons and new difficulties. He looks forward to college or university with pride, even though lessons grow harder and harder.

God's school of earthly life has in it all grades of advancement. Will you be a studious, courageous scholar and try to learn life's lessons well? It is such a wonderful thing to be a child of God, for that means to be an heir of God, an heir of His wisdom, His strength, His glory, His powers. "All things are yours," says Paul; "life, death, things present and things to come, all are yours, and ye are Christ's, and Christ is God's."

CHAPTER XIII.

SPECIAL PHYSIOLOGY.

With a feeling of reverence for ourselves we now take up the subject of special physiology to learn what makes us women. In the study of general physiology we find very few physical differences in the sexes, but when we come to investigate what is called the reproductive system we find entire difference of structure and of function.

Boys and girls in early childhood are much alike in their inclinations. They both love activity—to run, to climb, to shout, to laugh, to play. If left to themselves one sees not much more difference between boys and girls than between different individuals of the same sex. But as they grow and develop they begin to take on characteristics that indicate the evolution of sex.

The boy grows rapidly in height, his voice breaks, the signs of a moustache appear, he seems constrained and embarrassed in society, and yet he begins to show more politeness towards women and more of an inclination to be gallant to girls. He is becoming a man, and assumes manlike airs. Often, too, he becomes restless and willful, hard to govern, self-assertive, with an assumption of wisdom that provokes laughter from his elders. The boy is passing through a serious crisis and needs much wise and loving care. There are inner forces awakening that move him strangely; he does not understand himself, neither do his friends seem to understand him. Sometimes they snub and nag him, sometimes they tease and make fun of him. In either case he does not find home a happy place, and frequently leaves it to seek more sympathetic companionship elsewhere.

I once spoke to an audience of women and girls along this line, and appealed to the mothers and sisters to be kind to the boys in their homes who were between twelve and eighteen years of age, to remember that they were passing through the critical period of transition from boyhood to manhood, and to try and help them by sympathy and kindness. Some time later, as I was on the train, a young lady came and sat down by me and said: "I want to thank you for what you said to us the other day about boys. I have a brother about sixteen, and we have done just as you said; we have teased him about his moustache, and his voice, and his awkwardness, and laughed the more because it seemed to touch him. He had gotten so that he never would do anything for us girls, and we called him an old bear. Since I heard you I concluded that we had done wrong and I would make a change, so that evening I said kindly, 'Charlie, don't you want me to tie your cravat? I'd like to, ever so much.' I shall never forget the surprised look he gave me. It seemed as if he could not believe that I, his sister, wanted to do something to please him, but as soon as he saw I really meant it he accepted my offer with thanks, and since then it seems as if he could not do enough for me. Really I have almost cried to think that so little a thing would make him so grateful. I have invited him to go out with me several times, and he seems so glad to go. Then I've begun to make things for his room—little fancy things that I never thought a boy would care for—and he has appreciated them so much. Why, he even stays in his room sometimes, now, instead of going off with the boys. And the other day, when one of the boys came to see him, I heard him say, 'Come up and see my room,' and the other boy said, 'Well, I wish some one would fix up *my* room in such a jolly fashion.' Really," said the girl, "if you have done nothing on your trip but what you have done for me, in showing me how to be good to my brother, it has paid for you to come."

I often think of this little incident when I see boys at this critical age who are snubbed and teased just because they are leaving the land of boyhood to begin the difficult climb up the slopes of early manhood towards the grander height of maturity; and I wish all parents, sisters and older brothers would manifest a sympathy with the boy who, swayed by inner forces and influenced by outward temptation, is in a place of great danger.

The girl at this period is also passing through a crisis, but this fact is better understood by her friends than is the crisis of the boy's life. Her parents are anxious that she shall pass the crisis safely, and they have more patience with her eccentricities. She, too, often shows nervousness, irritability, petulance, or willfulness. She has headaches and backaches, she manifests lassitude and weariness, and is, perhaps, quite changed from her former self. She weeps easily or over nothing at all. She is dissatisfied with herself and the whole world. She feels certain vague, romantic longings that she could not explain if she tried. She inclines toward the reading of sensational love stories, and if not well instructed and self-respecting may be easily led into flirtations or conduct that later in life may make her blush to remember. Certain physical changes begin to be manifest. She increases rapidly in height, her figure grows fuller and more rounded, her breasts are often sore and tender. Hair makes its appearance on the body, and altogether she seems to be blossoming out into a fuller and riper beauty. She is changing from the girl to the woman, and this is a matter of sex. At this time the organs of sex, which have been dormant, awaken and take on their activity, and it is this awakening which is making itself felt throughout her whole organization.

We are sometimes apt to think that sex is located in certain organs only, but in truth sex, while centralized in the reproductive organs, makes itself manifest throughout the whole organization. I used to feel somewhat indignant when I heard people talk of sex in mind, and I boldly asserted that it did not exist, that intellect was neuter and had no reference to sex; but I do not feel so now. When I see what an influence the awakening of sex has upon the entire body and upon the character, I am led to believe that sex inheres in mind as well. That does not mean that the brain of one sex is either inferior or superior to the other; it means only that they differ; that men and women see things from different standpoints; that they are the two eyes of the race, and the use of both is needed to a clear understanding of any problem of human interest.

You know that the true perspective of objects cannot be had with one eye only, for each eye has its own range of vision, and one eye can see much farther on one side of an object than the other can. You can try this for yourself.

If, then, in viewing the vital problems of life we have the man's view only or the woman's view only, we have not the true perspective. We cannot say that either has superior powers of vision, but we can say that they differ, as this difference is inherent in them as men and women, and not merely as individuals.

Instead, then, of looking at sex as circumscribed, and perhaps as something low and vulgar, to be thought of and spoken of only with whispers or questionable mirth, we should see that sex is God's divinest gift to humanity, the power through which we come into the nearest likeness to Himself—the function by which we become creators and transmitters of our powers of body, mind, and soul.

It is important that a young woman should understand her own structure and the functions of all her organs, and so, with this feeling of reverence for sex, we will begin this study.

The trunk of the body is divided into three cavities; the upper or thoracic cavity contains the heart and lungs; the central or abdominal cavity contains the organs of nutrition, the stomach, liver, bowels, etc.; the lower or pelvic cavity contains two organs of elimination, the bladder and the rectum, and also the organs of reproduction, or of sex. Between the outlet of bladder and bowels is the inlet to the reproductive organs. This inlet is a narrow channel called the vagina, and is about six inches in length. At the upper end is the mouth of the womb or uterus. The words mean the same, but womb is Anglo-Saxon and *uterus* is Latin, and as Latin is the language of science, we will use that word. The uterus is the little nest or room in which the unborn baby has to live for three-fourths of a year. It is a small organ, about the size and shape of a small flattened pear. It is suspended with the small end downwards, and it is hollow. It is held in place by broad ligaments that extend outward to the sides, and by short, round ligaments from front to back. These ligaments do not hold it firmly in place, for it is necessary that it should be able to rise out of the pelvic into the abdominal cavity during pregnancy, as the baby grows too large to be contained in the small pelvic space.

On the posterior sides of the two broad ligaments are two small oval organs which are called ovaries, meaning the place of the eggs.

CHAPTER XIV.

BECOMING A WOMAN.

Perhaps you will remember that I once told you that all life is from an egg, the life of the plant, the fish, the bird, the human being. In the book "What a Young Girl Ought to Know" we discussed how all life originates in an egg, and why there must needs be fathers as well as mothers. We found that some eggs were small, were laid by the mothers in various places, and then left to develop or to die. Others were larger, covered with a large shell, and kept warm by the mothers sitting over them until the little ones were hatched. Others were so small that they developed in the mother's body until, as living creatures, they were born into the world. This is the case with the human being. He is first an egg in the mother's ovary. When this egg has reached a certain stage of development it passes from the ovary through a tube into the uterus. If it meets there, or on its way there, the fertilizing principle of the male, it remains there and develops into the child. If it does not meet this principle, it passes out through the vagina and is lost.

But the eggs, or ova—which is the Latin word meaning eggs—do not begin to ripen until the girl reaches the age of thirteen or fourteen, or, in other words, until she begins to become a woman. This passing away of the ovum (singular of ova) is called ovulation, and it occurs in the woman about every twenty-eight days. The uterus is lined by a mucous membrane similar to that which lines the mouth, and at this time of ovulation this membrane becomes swollen and soft, and little hemorrhages, or bleedings, occur for three or four days, the blood passing away through the vagina. This is called menstruation.

Sometimes, when girls have not been told beforehand of the facts of menstruation, they become greatly frightened at seeing this blood and imagine that they have some dreadful disease. If they have no friend to whom they can speak freely they sometimes do very injudicious things in their efforts to remove that which to them seems so strange and inexplicable. I have known of girls who washed their clothes in cold water and put them on wet, and so took cold and perhaps checked the menstrual flow, and as a consequence were injured for life, or may even have died years after as a result of this unwise conduct.

The girl who is wisely taught will recognize in this the outward sign of the fact that she has reached womanhood, that she has entered upon what is called the maternal period of a woman's life, the period when it is possible for her to become a mother.

This does not mean that she should become a mother while so young. It only means that the sex organs are so far developed that they are beginning to take up their peculiar functions. But they are like the immature buds of the flower, and need time for a perfect development. If she understands this, and recognizes her added value to the world through the perfecting of her entire organism, she will desire to take good care of herself, and during these years of early young womanhood to develop into all that is possible of sweetness, grace, purity, and all true womanliness.

Girls who are not wisely taught sometimes feel that this new physical function is a vexatious hindrance to their happiness. It is often accompanied with pain, and its periodical recurrence interferes with their plans for pleasure, and they in ignorance sometimes say, rebelliously, "O, I hate being a woman!"

A young woman once came to consult me professionally. She was a well-formed, good-looking girl, to all outward appearance lacking nothing in her physical make-up; but she was now twenty-two and had never menstruated, so she was aware that for some reason she was not like other girls. She came to ask me to make an examination and find out, if possible, what was wrong. She was engaged to be married, and knew that motherhood was in some way connected with menstruation, and she thought it might be possible that her physical condition would preclude the possibility of her becoming a mother, and, if so, it would be dishonorable to marry. Upon examination I discovered that all the organs of reproduction were lacking. When I disclosed this fact to her she exclaimed, with sadness, "Oh, why was I not made like other girls? I have heard them complain because they were girls, but I think if they were in my place, and knew that they could never have a home and children of their own, they would feel they had greater reason then to complain."

I think so, too. We seldom think of the fact that upon sex depend all the sweet ties of home and family. It is because of sex that we are fathers, mothers and children; that we have the dear family life, with its anniversaries of weddings and birthdays. It is through sex that the "desolate of the earth are set in families," and love and generosity have sway instead of selfishness. For this reason we ought to regard sex with reverent thought, to hold it sacred to the highest purposes, to speak of it ever with purest delicacy, and never with jesting or prurient smiles. I do not want you to center your thought on the physical facts of sex, but I would like to have you feel that womanhood, which is the mental, moral and physical expression of sex, is a glorious, divine gift, to be received with solemn thankfulness.

I want you, for the sake of a perfect womanhood, to take care of your bodily health, and yet I do not want you to feel that a woman must of necessity be a periodical semi-invalid.

CHAPTER XV.

ARTIFICIALITIES OF CIVILIZED LIFE.

Menstruation is a perfectly physiological process and should be without pain. Indeed, Dr. Mary Putnam Jacobi maintains that a woman ought to feel more life, vigor and ambition at that period than at any other time. As a fact, however, the majority of civilized women feel more or less lassitude and discomfort, and many suffer intensely. Whenever there is actual pain at any stage of the monthly period, it is because something is wrong, either in the dress, or the diet, or the personal and social habits of the individual. We certainly cannot believe that a kind and just God has made it necessary for women to suffer merely because they are women, and the observation of travelers among uncivilized peoples seems to indicate that where life is conducted according to nature's laws, the limitations of sex are less observable.

It is difficult for us to understand how very far our lives are from being natural. Professor Emmett, a world-renowned specialist in diseases peculiar to women, says: "At the very dawn of womanhood the young girl begins to live an artificial life utterly inconsistent with normal development. The girl of the period is made a woman before her time by associating too much with her elders, and in diet, dress, habits and tastes becomes at an early age but a reflection of her elder sisters. She may have acquired every accomplishment, and yet will have been kept in ignorance of the simplest features of her organization, and of the requirements for the preservation of her health. Her bloom is often as transient as that of the hothouse plant, where the flower has been forced by cultivation to an excess of development by stunting the growth of its branches and limiting the spread of its roots. A girl is scarcely in her teens before custom requires a change in her dress. Her shoulder-straps and buttons are given up for a number of strings about her waist and the additional weight of an increased length in skirt is added. She is unable to take the proper kind or necessary amount of exercise, even if she were not taught that it would be unladylike to make the attempt. Her waist is drawn into a shape little adapted to accommodate the organs placed there, and as the abdominal and spinal muscles are seldom brought into play they become atrophied. The viscera are thus compressed and displaced, and as the full play of the abdominal wall and the descent of the diaphragm are interfered with, the venous blood is hindered in its return to the heart."

Since Professor Emmett wrote this, public sentiment has changed, and it is no longer unladylike for girls to exercise; but with this increased freedom in custom should also come increased physical freedom through healthful clothing that allows perfect use of every muscle, more especially of the breathing muscles. I am sure you would rather pay out your money for that which shall add to your health and real happiness than to pay physicians to help you from suffering the just penalty of your own wrongdoing, and that is why I am anxious to give you this needed instruction. I do not care to have you study much about diseases, but I want you to understand very fully how, through care of yourself, to prevent disease.

CHAPTER XVI.

SOME CAUSES OF PAINFUL MENSTRUATION.

There should be no pain at menstruation, but that pain is quite common cannot be denied. Let us look for other causes than are found in the dress.

One frequent cause is found in the ignorance of girls, and their consequent injudicious conduct at the time of the beginning of sexual activity. At this time of life the girl is often called lazy because she manifests lassitude, and this is nature's indication that she should rest. The vital forces are busy establishing a new function, and the energy that has been expressed in bodily activity is now being otherwise employed. The girl who has been properly brought up, whose muscles are strong, and whose nervous supply is abundant, may have no need of especial care at this time, but the average girl needs much judicious care, in order that her physical womanhood shall be healthfully established. She should be guarded from taking cold, from overexertion, from social dissipation, and especially from mental excitement, and other causes of nervousness. I would like to call your attention to the great evil of romance-reading, both in the production of premature development and in the creation of morbid mental states which will tend to the production of physical evils, such as nervousness, hysteria, and a host of maladies which largely depend upon disturbed nerves.

Girls are not apt to understand the evils of novel-reading, and may think it is only because mothers have outlived their days of romance that they object to their daughters enjoying such sentimental reading; but the wise mother understands the effects of sensational reading upon the physical organization, and wishes to protect her daughter from the evils thus produced.

It is not only that novel-reading engenders false and unreal ideas of life, but the descriptions of love-scenes, of thrilling, romantic episodes, find an echo in the girl's physical system and tend to create an abnormal excitement of her organs of sex, which she recognizes only as a pleasurable mental emotion, with no comprehension of the physical origin or the evil effects.

Romance-reading by young girls will, by this excitement of the bodily organs, tend to create their premature development, and the child becomes physically a woman months, or even years, before she should.

In one case it became my duty to warn a girl of eleven, who was an omnivorous reader of romances, that such reading was in all probability hastening her development, and she would become a woman in bodily functions while she ought yet to be a child. Her indications of approaching womanhood were very apparent. By becoming impressed by my words she gave up romance-reading, devoted herself to outdoor sports, to nature studies, and the vital forces diverted from the reproductive system were employed in building up her physical energy, her health improved, her nervousness disappeared, and three years later her function of menstruation was painlessly established.

A frequent cause of painful menstruation is found in habitual neglect of the bowels. The evils of constipation are common to the majority of women and girls, and the foundation is laid in childhood. Mothers are not careful enough in instructing children in the need of care in this respect, and so the habit is formed early in life, and the results are felt later.

If the bowels are not evacuated regularly the matter to be cast out of the body accumulates in the rectum and large bowel, and by pressure the circulation of the blood is impeded and congestion ensues. This extends to all the pelvic organs; the uterus and ovaries thus congested will soon manifest disease, and painful menstruation be the result.

One of the most frequent causes of pain is congestion produced by displacements. People are very apt to think that the displacement of the uterus is the main factor, but in my opinion it is a secondary condition, and not the one to be first considered. The uterus is a small organ, not vital to the individual, is very movable, and not sensitive, so that its displacement alone could hardly be considered sufficient to cause so great a train of evils as is frequently manifest. But the liver, stomach and bowels are large, vital organs, and their displacement leads to greater consequences. You learned at school that the bowels are over twenty feet in length, weigh as much as twelve or fifteen pounds, are supported in a way that makes it possible for them to sag into the abdominal cavity and press upon the pelvic organs. Dr. Emerson, of the Boston School of Oratory, asserts that in most adults the stomach and bowels are from two to six inches below their normal location; and, as I have said before, Dr. Kellogg often finds the stomach lying in the abdominal cavity as low down as the umbilicus. What has caused this sagging of the abdominal viscera? They certainly must have been intended to keep their place unless there has been some interference. We find just such interference in the ordinary arrangement of the clothing. Tight waists and bands, and skirts supported by the hips, are cause sufficient for these displacements.

Just above the hips there is no bony structure to protect and support the soft, muscular parts. They yield to pressure, and the internal viscera, deprived of muscular support, sink until they rest on the pelvic organs. If, when you look at your abdomen, you see depressions or hollows on each side below the floating ribs, you may know that the bowels have sagged down out of place. If you feel great weariness, backache, or a dragged down feeling in standing or walking, you may know that the contents of the abdomen are pulling on their attachments or pressing on the pelvic organs. Thus displaced, circulation is hindered and the organs all become congested, or filled with blood that moves very slowly. This congested condition is increased at menstruation, and great pain may result.

It is well to have the counsel of some good, honest physician under such circumstances, but should you be where it is not possible to have such counsel, you may still be able to do something to help yourself. In the first place, you can rearrange your clothing so as to relieve all the organs from external weight or pressure, and, in the second place, you can support the abdominal walls by applying pressure from below. I have known cases of painful menstruation entirely relieved by simply supporting the bowels by a bandage, thus relieving the uterus of pressure and allowing a free circulation through all the internal organs.

A very simple and practical bandage can be made at home at almost no cost, either in time or money. Buy some thin, cheap cotton flannel. Take lengthwise of the goods a strip long enough to go around the body at the hips, which will be a yard or a little over, and wide enough to fit from the thighs up to the waist, perhaps eight inches. Put darts on the sides and in the center of the back, to make it fit the figure. Make a couple of straps four inches wide and half a yard long; cut off one end of each diagonally. Sew these slanting ends to the lower side of the band about four inches from the center, that is eight inches apart, and so that the short side of the strap will be towards the center. Do not hem either band or straps, but overcast them; then they will not feel uncomfortable.

In order to adjust the band properly it will be well to lie down on the back upon the bandage with the knees raised. Press the hands low down upon the abdomen and raise the contents. Repeat this several times; then draw the bandage around, pin with safety pins, draw the straps up between the limbs and fasten with safety pins to the bandage. The support thus given is found to be very comfortable, and girls who have much trouble in walking or standing during their menstrual periods would find this simple bandage a great help at that time.

When the bandage is removed at night you should rub and manipulate the abdominal walls so as to increase the circulation and stimulate in them a better circulation and thus make you stronger.

By deep breathing in a proper standing attitude the abdominal viscera are lifted upward, and if the firmness of the abdominal walls is at the same time increased by exercise, the difficulties may be largely overcome. Some exercises will be found in Chapter XXIII. which are calculated to strengthen the walls and to lift the internal organs.

I wish to call your attention to a cause of displacement that is quite generally overlooked, and that is, a wrong attitude.

Dr. Eliza Mosher has made a very thorough study of this matter, and she says that the common habit of standing on one foot is productive of marked deformities of both face and body and of serious displacements of internal organs. It is seldom a girl or woman can be found whose body is perfectly symmetrical. By standing on one foot, the hip and shoulder of one side approach each other, and so lessen the space within the abdomen on that side. On the other side a support has been removed for the contents of the abdomen, and they sag down until they pry the uterus out of place and press it over towards the side where there is less pressure. The broad ligament on one side is stretched from use and on the other side shortened from disuse, and so the uterus remains permanently dislocated.

Dr. Mosher thinks that standing continually with the weight on the left foot is more injurious than bearing it on the right foot, for it causes the uterus and ovaries to press upon the rectum and so produces a mechanical constipation, especially during menstruation.

Wrong habits of sitting will produce the same results. If the girl sits at school with one elbow on the desk, the head will be turned to the opposite side and the spine will be inclined from the perpendicular, and a lateral curvature be likely to result. If she carries her books always on the same side, it will tend to increase the curvature. If she sits with both elbows supported, her shoulders will be pushed up. If her body is twisted as she sits, a strain comes upon the muscles, and some ligaments will be lengthened and others shortened, thus producing a lateral curvature.

To sit "on the small of the back," that is, slipping down in the chair, bracing the shoulders against the chair-back, tends to injure the nerves by pressure, and also to create a posterior curvature of the spine.

Does it not seem unfortunate that we should allow ourselves even to form such wrong habits of sitting and standing? And now we ask, How shall we know when we are in a correct attitude?

We have comparatively few correct examples to imitate. I notice people everywhere, and I see that old and young stand incorrectly. The head is poked forward, the shoulders are rounded, the chest is flattened, and the curve in the lower part of the back is straightened. The whole figure is out of balance, and therefore not harmonious. Not only is the beauty of the figure destroyed, but the internal organs are displaced. Many a mother who sees her daughter thus growing round-shouldered keeps telling her to throw her shoulders back; but to follow this command only increases the difficulty. The shoulders are not primarily at fault, but the trouble originates in non-use of the front waist muscles. These muscles, weakened by disease because of tight clothing and corset steels, and also by cramped positions in school or at work, refuse to hold the body erect, and it "lops" just at this point. This "lopping" disturbs the harmonious relation of the weights of shoulders, abdomen, head, and the large lower gluteal muscles with which nature has cushioned the lower part of the body, and so they are obliged to readjust themselves to balance each other, and the awkward, ungainly, unhealthful posture results.

What is needed is to restore the right relation of these weights and all will again be harmonious. Do not interfere with the shoulders, but straighten the front of the body by elevating the chest and raising the head until it is supported directly on the spine, letting the shoulders take care of themselves. If the abdomen is now held back and the gluteal muscles raised, the beautiful curves of the spine will be restored, the shoulders will be straightened, and the internal organs will have a chance to resume their natural position.

A very easy way of finding out if you have the correct attitude is to place your toes against the bottom of the door. Now bring your chest up to touch the door, and throw the lower part of the spine backward so that there will be a space between the abdomen and the door. Place the head erect, with the chin drawn in towards the neck, and you will have very nearly the correct attitude. It may seem a little tiresome at first, because you will be apt to hold yourself in position with needless tension of muscles, but you will soon learn to relax the unnecessary tension, and then you will find the position the most comfortable possible. You can walk farther without fatigue, and stand longer without backache, because the body is placed in the attitude in which all parts occupy their designed relation to each other.

One very important fact is that in the wrong attitude the abdominal organs crowd down into the pelvis, while in the correct position they are supported and kept from sagging, so that the matter of a correct attitude is not only a matter of beauty, but also of health.

In sitting, also, the most comfortable posture is the most healthful; that is, with the body squarely placed on the seat, and equally supported upon the pelvis—not leaning back against the chair, unless the chair should chance to be so constructed that it supports the lower part of the back and keeps the body erect.

CHAPTER XVII.

"FEMALE DISEASES."

We hear a great deal in these days of "female diseases," by which is meant the displacements of the organs of the reproductive system; that is, of the uterus, ovaries, etc. These displacements are many, for the uterus may not only drop down out of place, but it may be tipped towards one side or the other, to the front or the back; or it may be bent upon itself in various directions. These different displacements cause much pain, and often result in ulcerations and profuse discharges which are known as the "whites," or scientifically as leucorrhea.

I only mention these things incidentally, so that I may call your attention to the things you may do to prevent them.

A great many girls and women are spending large sums of money in being doctored for these difficulties who need not suffer with them at all if they had known how to dress healthfully; and many are bearing much anxiety over the possibility of becoming sufferers with these distressing diseases who could have their burden of fear removed by the knowledge that "female diseases," in the great majority of cases, are the results of wrong habits of dress and life. Leucorrhea is not a disease. It is a symptom of abnormal conditions, and to be cured it is needful that the conditions shall be understood.

Dr. Kellogg says, "Leucorrhea may result from simple congestion of the bloodvessels of the vaginal mucous membrane, due to improper dress. It may also be occasioned by taking cold, and by a debilitated condition of the stomach."

Leucorrhea is merely an abnormal increase of a normal secretion. All mucous membrane secretes mucus in small quantities—enough to keep the membrane moist. When from any cause this secretion is increased, we have what is called a catarrhal condition. As all cavities that communicate with the air are lined with mucous membrane, this catarrhal condition may exist in the nose, the throat, the eyes, the ears, the bowels, or the reproductive organs, and will be named according to the location.

A natural increase of this secretion takes place just before and after menstruation, and should occasion no anxiety, but if continued during the remainder of the month, especially if very profuse, of offensive odor, or bloody in character, it needs the attention of the skilled physician.

I do not wish to make you think constantly of yourself as diseased, and so I do not give you directions as to local self-treatment. Many symptoms can be overcome by general care of the health-habits of the girl, and if they do not yield to this general care it is better to consult a responsible physician than to tamper with yourself.

And here let me give you a word of warning. If you need medical care, never consult the traveling doctors who advertise to do such wonderful things. They charge big fees and give a little medicine and then move on, and you have no redress if they have not accomplished all that they have promised. They live off the gullibility of people. Again, never take patent medicines. Wonderful discoveries, favorite prescriptions and the like may be harmless, and they may not. And even if they are, how can you judge that they are suited to your special case? That they cured some one else is not proof that they will benefit you, and you run a risk by taking them as an experiment. One very serious danger in the taking of patent medicines is the fact that they are so largely alcoholic in composition, and girls and women have all too often been led into the alcohol habit and become habitual drunkards through taking some advertised remedy.

Another has correctly said: "If you need the consultation and advice of a physician go to your family physician, or, if you prefer, go to some other physician; but always select one whose moral character and acknowledged ability render him a suitable and safe adviser in such a time of need. Above all things avoid quacks. The policy they pursue is to frighten you, to work upon your imagination, and to make such alarming and unreliable statements as will induce you to purchase their nostrums and subject yourself to such a series of humiliations and impositions as will enable them to pilfer your purse and without rendering you in return any value received, but likely leave you in a much worse condition than they found you."

You will probably be advised by your personal friends, who may know of your ailments, to take hot douches, and perhaps you may wonder why I do not prescribe them for leucorrhea, and kindred difficulties.

I do not commend them for the fact that I do not want you to be turning your constantly anxious thought towards yourself in these matters. If you need such treatment, let it be prescribed by your physician, who knows exactly your condition. As far as possible turn your thoughts from the reproductive system. Take care of your general health, dress properly, obey all the rules of hygiene in regard to diet, sleep, bathing, special cleanliness, and care, and then forget as far as possible the physical facts of womanhood.

An excellent addition to your general bathing can be taken once a week in the form of a sitz bath, which is effective for cleanliness, and also for the reduction of congestion. If you have no sitz bath-tub, an ordinary wash-tub can be made to answer by raising one side an inch or two by means of some support. Have the water at a comfortable temperature, say about 98 degrees, and if you have no thermometer you can gauge the heat by putting in three gallons of cold water and add one gallon of boiling water. Sit down in the tub and cover yourself with a blanket. In about ten minutes add by degrees a gallon of cold water. Remain sitting a minute or two longer, then rub dry.

Many people are afraid to use cold water after hot, in bathing, for fear they will take cold, but that is just the way to prevent such a result from the hot bath. The hot water has caused all the pores on the surface of the body to open, and the bodily heat is rapidly lost through this cause. The cold water, quickly applied, causes the pores to close, leaves the skin in a tonic condition, and conserves the bodily heat. One should never take a hot bath without following it with a *quick* cold application to the surface. It should continue, however, but for a moment.

This kind of a bath is very useful for all chronic congestions of the abdominal and pelvic viscera, such as piles, constipation, painful menstruation, leucorrhea, or other affections of the reproductive organs. It is also very helpful in headaches due to congestion of the brain. If there is too little blood in the brain it might produce wakefulness, but when the brain is too full of blood this bath tends to produce sound and refreshing sleep.

A foot bath may be taken at the same time as the sitz bath, and in this case the water should be warmer than that in the sitz bath, and as the person rises from the sitz bath she should step into it, so that her feet will get the tonic effect of the cold water.

The average age at which menstruation first appears is fourteen, but some girls menstruate as early as eleven, while others may not develop till some years later. Frequently, when the girl does not manifest this symptom of womanly development, the mother becomes anxious and begins to give forcing medicines. She knows that girls often die with consumption in their early young womanhood, and has heard that it was because they did not physically develop, and she fears that such danger threatens her daughter, and imagines that if something can be done to "bring on her courses," as she expresses it, the danger will be averted.

In this case she has reversed cause and effect. The consumptive girl did not menstruate because she had not the vitality to do so. The consumption was the cause, the non-menstruation the effect. To produce hemorrhage from the reproductive system by strong, forcing medicines is only to increase the danger. The only thing to do is to improve the general health, and if the girl can increase in strength until she has more vital force than suffices to keep her alive, the function that is vital—not to her, but to the race—will establish itself.

The failure of the menses to appear at the average age may be due merely to a slow development, and in this case there is nothing to do but wait. If the girl seems well, if she has no backache, no headache, no general lassitude, no undue nervous symptoms, the mere non-appearance of the menses need occasion no alarm. If, however, she has these symptoms, it is an evidence that nature is attempting to establish the function and is hindered either by general lack of vitality or by some local condition, and in either case the giving of forcing medicines would be a mistake. The weekly sitz bath would do no harm as a semi-local measure. All proper precautions should be observed as to maintenance of general health and mental serenity, and if these do not prove sufficient the physician should be consulted.

In the case I mentioned, where the reproductive organs were lacking, the girl had been subjected to a long course of home medication which had proven disastrous to her digestion, and yet, as will be readily understood, had not resulted in the establishment of a function that is dependent upon organs which, in this case, did not exist.

Sometimes there are slight mechanical hindrances which can only be determined by the physician, though their presence will be indicated by the symptoms of menstruation without the accompanying sanguineous discharge. In these cases the home medication is dangerous. If the girl regularly has symptoms of approaching menstruation, with pain and bloating, and these subside without flow, it would be wise to consult the physician instead of resorting to domestic remedies or letting the matter go on without attention.

Quite frequently the first appearance of menstruation is followed by weeks or even months of freedom from its reappearance. In these cases no alarm need be felt as long as the general health is not affected. Again, there may be suspension of the function from change of surroundings. Girls who go away to school often suffer from irregularity. I have known of a case where the girl never menstruated during the school year, but was perfectly regular during vacations.

These cases may be accounted for by the nervous strain, the using up of vital forces in mental effort to such degree that there is nothing left with which to carry on the menstrual function. In all such cases it is wise to watch carefully the general health, and if all functions are not properly conducted, to reduce the strain until the vitality is able to keep all functions in order.

Girls are sometimes disturbed because the flow is scanty, and think they should do something to increase the amount. It is no doubt true that profuse menstrual flow is the result of our artificial lives. If we lived more normally we should have naturally a scanty menstrual flow. Therefore if a girl has good health and no monthly pain and the flow is scanty, she may consider herself as more nearly in a normal state, and be thankful.

If, however, the menses are suddenly less than normal it denotes a suppression, which may be the result of cold, exhaustion of body, weariness of nerves, mental anxiety, or disturbance of the emotions.

If gradual suppression occurs, accompanied by loss of health, it indicates some constitutional difficulty or local trouble which demands professional counsel.

Profuse menstruation is also a relative term, as there is no definite standard as to amount of menstrual flow, nor the length of time it should continue. The profuseness must be measured by the condition of the individual. Where health seems fully maintained there would appear no cause for anxiety. But if there is a marked increase over the amount usual for the individual, if great weakness and prostration is produced, either at the time or afterward, it may be called profuse, and the cause may be either debility, that is weakness, or plethora, which means fullness. If from the latter, there will be throbbing headache, pain in the back, and general signs of fever. If from debility, there will be pallor, weakness, and perhaps an almost continuous flow.

As may be imagined, the treatment in the two cases will differ. The full-blooded girl should be put on a plain, unstimulating diet, with plenty of out-door exercise during the month, but about twenty-four hours before the flow is expected she should have complete mental and physical rest. She should remain in bed, and apply cold wet cloths over the abdomen and between the thighs for an hour at a time, with intervals of at least one-half hour between the applications. The bowels should be freed from all fecal matter, and cool, small enemas be given two or three times a day. If these simple measures do not avail, the doctor should be consulted.

The pale and debilitated girl needs to rest. Sometimes, if hemorrhage continues almost from one period to the next, she should remain in bed even after the flow seems checked. The great desideratum is to build up the general health, not by tonics, which are usually only stimulants, but by the judicious observance of the laws of health. This will, in many cases, call for the advice of the physician, who can see and study the patient and her special conditions. It is not safe to trust to book-doctoring.

CHAPTER XVIII.

CARE DURING MENSTRUATION.

I have said that I do not want you to think yourself a semi-invalid and so be "fussy" about yourself, but I have also said that I want you to take care of yourself at all times, and especially during your menstrual periods. How can you make these ideas agree with each other?

I know that many writers say that a girl should spend one day each month in bed, or at least lying down; that there are some things that should always be forbidden to girls, simply because they are girls, such as running up and down stairs. These wholesale restrictions make girls rebellious at their womanhood. I simply want you to use good sense at all times in your care of yourself.

Knowing the fact that just before and during menstruation the uterus is heavier than at other times, because engorged with blood, and remembering that it is loosely suspended, it is easy to understand that long walks or severe exercise at the menstrual period will more easily cause it to sag, and this sagging becoming permanent may cause pain, backache, and other discomforts. Therefore, having good sense, you will not plan to take long rides or walks or do any severe exercise. At the same time moderate exercise in proper clothing will tend to relieve pelvic congestion by equalizing the circulation, and if the clothing is properly adjusted and the muscles are strong and well-developed, an ordinary amount of physical activity may be beneficial rather than harmful.

Girls are so often told that they must not walk at their monthly periods, must not study, must not ride, etc., etc., that it really is no wonder that they feel it a very undesirable thing to be a woman. My observation leads me to believe that if girls from earliest childhood were dressed loosely, with no clothing suspended on the hips, if their muscles were well developed through judicious exercise, they would seldom find it necessary to be semi-invalids at any time. In fact, we do sometimes find a young woman who has no

What a Young Woman Ought to Know

consciousness of physical disturbance during menstruation. She can pursue her usual avocations without hindrance, and finds her physical womanhood no bar to any enjoyment.

This is as it should be; but as girls have not all been well developed and properly dressed, we cannot assert that all girls can be indifferent to physical conditions at this time. If a girl is well, has no pain or discomfort, then I would say, let her use good common sense in the ordering of her daily life and give the matter no special or anxious thought. If she has pain or uneasiness, let her govern her life accordingly, using care, taking some rest at the time of the menses; but, above all things, let her arrange her clothing at all times so as to secure for herself absolute freedom of movement. Then let her, during the intervals between the menstrual periods, endeavor by judicious exercise to build up strong muscular structure around the vital organs, such structure as will support the *viscera* where they belong, and in time she will probably find herself growing free from menstrual pain.

During the painful periods resulting from congestion it is often advisable to keep the recumbent position, and to use heat both externally and internally. However, I would advise never using alcoholic beverages. Their apparent usefulness lies principally in the hot water with which they are administered, and the danger of forming the alcohol habit is too great to justify their use.

There are cases of nervous pain at menstruation that are aggravated by heat and diminished by cold. I knew such a case where a girl at school, suffering with menstrual pain, alarmed teachers and friends by wringing towels out of cold water and laying them over her abdomen. But the alarm subsided when they saw that the pain soon passed away under the cold application. The girl was one in whom there were no local congestions, but great nervous exhaustion and heat always increased her sufferings, while cold allayed.

I have read that a woman should not bathe or change her underwear while menstruating. I cannot see how soiled clothing can be more healthful than that which is clean; and if well-aired, I should no more object to your putting on clean underwear than to your changing your dress. Most especially would I advise a frequent change of napkins, in order to remove those which are soiled from their irritating contact with the body. A full bath during menstruation would, for most people, be unadvisable, but the cleansing of the private parts is imperative. For this, tepid water, with good soap, may be used daily or oftener. Other parts of the body may be rubbed with a wet cloth, followed by vigorous, dry rubbing. Cleanliness at all times is certainly a mark of refinement.

You should use good sense and not run out in thin slippers on wet or cold ground; but if your feet get wet through accident, keep in motion until you can make a change of shoes and stockings. There is little danger from wet feet to those in good health, if they keep in vigorous motion.

As to other rules, they are those that pertain to the care of health at all times: loose clothing, deep breathing, wholesome food, plenty of sleep, sunlight, pure air, exercise according to your strength, and, above all, serenity of mind, accepting the fact of physical womanhood, together with a recognition of its sacredness and dignity.

As a minor item, I would suggest that the napkins be fastened to straps that go over the shoulder and are then joined together in front and back to an end piece, on each of which a button is sewn. Buttonholes in the napkins at the corners, diagonal from each other, will make them easily attached or removed. The napkins should be of a material that is quickly absorbent of the flow. Cheesecloth is cheap, and can be burned or otherwise disposed of after using. It may be protected by an outer strip of unbleached muslin which is almost water-proof.

A very comfortable way of arranging napkins that are to be used from time to time is to take a piece of linen or cotton diaper sixteen inches square. About three inches from one end, make on each side an incision four inches long. Fold this strip in the middle lengthwise, and sew together up to the end of the incisions. This makes a band with a sort of pocket in the middle. Hem the cut edges. Fold the napkin over, four inches on each side, that is as deep as the incisions. Then fold crosswise until you can enclose the whole in the pocket in the band. This makes a thick center and thin ends by which to attach the napkin to the suspender.

I hold that mental serenity is one of the essentials of healthful menstrual periods, and this cannot be had if the mind is continually troubled and the thought centered on the physical condition. I would be glad to have your mind freed from the ideas of sex matters as far as possible. It is a scientific fact that thinking continually of an organ tends to disturb that organ. I know a man who was so afraid of heart disease that he felt of his pulse every few minutes and kept a stethoscope on the head of his bed to listen to his heart in the night. I would have been surprised had he not had heart trouble.

CHAPTER XIX.

SOLITARY VICE.

As the reproductive system awakens to activity it naturally attracts the attention of the girl, and an effort should be made to call her thoughts to other themes.

As I have said before, the reading of sensational love stories is most detrimental. The descriptions of passionate love scenes arouse in the reader a thrill through her own sexual organism that tends to increase its activity and derange its normal state. Girls often mature into women earlier than they should, because through romances, through jests of associates in regard to beaus and lovers, and through indulgence in sentimental fancies their sexual systems are unduly stimulated and aroused. This stimulation sometimes leads to the formation of an evil habit, known as self-abuse. The stimulation of the sex organs is accompanied with a pleasurable sensation, and this excitement may be created by mechanical means, or even by thought. Many girls who are victims of this most injurious habit are unaware of its dangers, although they instinctively feel that they do not want it known. Others who would not stoop to a mechanical exciting of themselves do so through thoughts, and do not know that they are just as truly guilty of self-abuse as the girl who uses the hand or other mechanical means.

The results of self-abuse are most disastrous. It destroys mental power and memory, it blotches the complexion, dulls the eye, takes away the strength, and may even cause insanity. It is a habit most difficult to overcome, and may not only last for years, but in its tendency be transmitted to one's children.

If you have from the first thought nobly of yourself, you will have fallen into no such debasing habit. But if, through ignorance, you have acquired it, how shall you overcome it?

I should hesitate to write more on this subject did I not know that many girls fall victims to this evil through ignorance, and many who thus fall could and would have been saved had they been rightly instructed. I therefore desire that you shall be wise.

Every normal function of the body is attended with a pleasurable sensation. We enjoy eating, seeing, walking. Odors bring sensations which are agreeable, the sense of touch may give pleasure, and as we enjoy these sensations in fact, so we may enjoy them in memory or in imagination. We can recall the beauty of the rose, the perfume of the mignonette, the flavor of the orange, or we can imagine new combinations of these delights. We feel joy or grief through reading vivid descriptions, or we can ourselves create imaginary scenes in which we are actors, who suffer or enjoy.

The reproductive system is the seat of great nervous susceptibility, and the excitation of these nerves gives a pleasurable sensation. This excitation may be thought a local mechanical irritation or it may be mental. In little children it may be caused by lack of cleanliness of the external organs. An irritation is produced, and an attempt to allay this by rubbing produces an agreeable feeling, which may be repeated until the evil habit of self-abuse is formed.

Sometimes constipation, by creating a pelvic congestion, will have the same result. Sometimes clothing which is too small may, by undue pressure on the parts, call the thought of the child to these organs, and in an attempt to remove the pressure by pulling the clothing away the habit may be begun.

Sometimes the tiny pin-worms in the rectum may wander into the vagina, and the little girl feel a constant annoyance, which rubbing allays temporarily, but which results in the evil habit of the use of the hands to produce an agreeable sensation. Thus through avoidable causes the evil habit may be acquired. Then it may be taught by one thus learning it to another who, without this instruction, would never have acquired it.

But new dangers arise as the girl approaches the age when the reproductive system begins to take on the activity that indicates approaching womanhood. The normal congestion of the parts causes a hitherto unknown consciousness of sex, and unless she is warned she may at this period acquire the habit without knowing its evils.

All functions necessary to the preservation of the individual life are attended with pleasure, and so are those which are for the continuation of the species. While the emotion may be pleasurable, it is at the same time the most exhausting, that can be experienced. We see that in some forms of animal existence parenthood is purchased at the expense of the life of the parent; and while in the human being the procreative act does not kill, it exhausts, and no doubt takes from the vital force of those exercising it. One can feel justified to lose a part of her own life if she is conferring life upon others, but to indulge in such a waste of vital force merely for pleasure is certainly never excusable, and least excusable of all is the arousing of pleasurable emotions by a direct violation of natural law.

The only natural method of arousing a recognition of sexual feeling is as God has appointed in holy marriage, and the self-respecting girl feels that no approach of personal familiarity is either right or proper. But it may be that she does not know that feelings may be awakened by the imagination which are as wrong morally as, and more injurious physically than, actual deeds, and so may allow her mind to revel in fancies that would shock her as actualities.

I received a letter not long ago from a young woman who most emphatically asserted that she would never, never, never permit familiarities, and then most innocently says, "but it wouldn't be wrong to imagine yourself enjoying the embrace of some certain one, would it?"

It is just this idea that there is no wrong in thought that weakens virtue's fortress and renders it easily demolished. Girls who would shrink from use of mechanical means to arouse sexual desire will permit themselves to revel in imaginary scenes of love-making with real or unreal individuals, or in mental pictures which arouse the spasmodic feelings of sexual pleasure, and yet be unaware that they are guilty of self-abuse.

Sexual feeling in itself is not base, but it can be debased either in thought or in deed. Rightly considered, it is the indication of the possession of the most sacred powers, that of the perpetuation of life.

"Passion is the instinct for preservation of one's kind, the voice of the life principle, the sign of creative power." These last four words open before us a wonderful field of thought. "Creative power!" What does that mean? Is creative power limited to reproduction of kind? Do you not create when you work out with brain some idea and then embody it in some visible form? Worth is said to create an artistic dress, the actor creates his part in the play, the musician creates the arrangement of harmonies which are represented in musical signs, and in the same sense you may be in a myriad of ways a creator.

With the beginning of activity of sexual life in yourself came increased development and new energy, beauty, and power, and the preservation and right use of that life will continue to be a source of power. "When the signs of this creative power come throbbing and pulsing in every fiber, it only shows that one has more and greater ability to create than ever before. One knows by this that she can now do greater work than she has done or is doing;" so says one writer.

Is it not a beautiful thought that this feeling, which we have supposed we must fight as something low, is in reality the stirring of a divine impulse which we can control and govern and make to serve us in all high and noble deeds?

If you hold such noble thoughts in your heart concerning yourself, you will need no threatenings to keep you from self-debasement and self-defilement. You will not need to be told of the loss of physical strength or of beauty, of memory or of reason, through evil habits of solitary vice, for they will have no temptation for you, even as you do not need threats of police and prisons to keep you from stealing, because honesty is the active and guiding principle of your life.

But supposing you have already acquired the evil habit and are now awakened to the wrong you are doing yourself; you observe the lack of lustre in the eye, the sallow, blotched complexion; you realize your loss of nerve-power manifested in cold and clammy hands, backache, lassitude, irritability, lack of memory, and inability to concentrate thought. What shall you do to overcome and to gain control of yourself? The question is a serious one, for no habit is more tyrannical than the dominion of unrestrained sexual desire. Its victims often fight for years, only to be conquered at last. If there was no cure but in fighting, I should feel that the case was almost hopeless.

The very first thing to do is to change the mental attitude in regard to the whole matter of sex; to hold it in thought as sacred, holy, consecrated to the highest of all functions, that of procreation. Recognize that, conserved and controlled, it becomes a source of energy to the individual. Cleanse the mind of all polluting images by substituting this purer thought; then go to work to establish correct habits of living in dress, diet, exercise, etc. See to it that there are no such causes of pelvic congestions as prolapsed bowels, caused by tight clothing or constipation; keep the skin active; and, above all, keep the mind healthfully occupied.

The victim of self-abuse has, through the frequent repetition of the habit, built up an undue amount of brain that is sensitive to local irritation of the sex-organs or to mental pictures of sex-pleasure. She must now allow this part of the brain to become quiescent, and she should go to work to build up other brain centers. Let her train her sight by close observation of form, color, size, location. Let her cultivate her sense of hearing in the study of different qualities of sound, tone, pitch, intensity, duration, timbre; her sense of touch, by learning to judge with closed eyes of different materials, of quality of fiber, of the different degrees of temperature, of roughness or smoothness, of density; in fact, let her endeavor to become alert, observant, along all the lines of sense-perception. Let her study nature, leaf-forms, cloud-shapes, insects, flowers, birds, bird-songs, the causes of natural phenomena; and, above all, let her keep out of the realm of the artificial, the sentimental, the emotional, and, holding firmly to the thought that creative energy is symbolized by desire and can be dignified and consecrated to noblest purposes, she will find herself daily growing into a stronger, more beautiful self-control.

CHAPTER XX.

BE GOOD TO YOURSELF.

I witnessed the other day a parting between two men. The elder, as he took the younger by the hand, said, "Good-by, my boy; be good to yourself;" and the younger responded, heartily, "Oh, there is no danger but I'll be that." I wondered, as I saw the laughing face, so full of the indications of the love of pleasure, if he really would be good to himself, or if he would interpret it to mean to indulge himself in all kinds of sensuous gratification. It is a great thing to be truly good to one's self, and I would give the injunction with the highest ideal. Be good to your real self with that true goodness that sees the end from the beginning, that realizes the tendency of certain forms of pleasure, and that claims the privilege of being master of the senses, and not their slave.

"Well," you say, rather deprecatingly, "you can't expect young people to act as staid and wise as you old folks. We want some fun." So you do, and that is perfectly right. You should want fun and have fun. All I ask is that you shall try to understand what real, true fun is.

I have seen young folks pull the chair from under some one "for fun," and the result was pain and perhaps permanent injury to the object of the joke.

I have known young men to imagine they were having "fun" when they went on a spree, to get "gloriously drunk," as they phrased it. You can see no fun in this. You realize that it is a most serious tragedy, with not an element of real fun in it, involving, as it does, the loss of health, the risking of life, the possibility of crime, the heart-break of friends, and perhaps even death. It is altogether a wrong idea of fun.

I have known girls in the secrecy of their rooms to smoke cigarettes "for fun," and in that I am sure that you see no amusement. It was a lowering of the standard of womanhood; it was tampering with a poison; it was something to be ashamed of, rather than something to call fun.

I have known young men and women to enter into flirtations "for fun." I knew a girl whose chief delight seemed to be in getting young men in love with her, only to cast them aside when tired of their adoration. She called this fun, but it was cruelty. In olden times men amused themselves by throwing Christians to wild beasts and watching them while being torn to pieces. This was their idea of fun, and the flirt's idea of amusement seems to be of the same order. She plays with the man as the cat with the mouse, and experiences no pangs of conscience when, torn and bleeding in heart, she tosses him aside for a new victim.

There are other young people who would not enter into such serious flirtations, and yet are unduly familiar with each other. They mean nothing by their endearments and familiarities, and neither will suffer any pangs when the pleasant intimacy is ended. Can we not call this innocent fun? They have indulged in some unobserved hand-pressures, or a few stolen kisses; but neither believed the other to mean anything serious. It was only fun; what harm could there be in that?

Many girls to-day are reasoning thus, and many of these may pass through the experience without loss of reputation; they may subsequently marry honorably, and become respected and beloved mothers. But ask any of these girls, in her mature years, when her own daughters are growing up around her, if she wants them to pass through the same experiences. I once knew a beautiful young woman who thought it was fun to have these familiar intimacies with young men, because, as she said, she knew how far to go. I saw her in her maturity, with daughters of her own, and heard her say that when she recalled her own girlish escapades, even in the darkness of the night the blushes would rush over her from head to foot, and in heartfelt agony she would say to herself, "Oh, I wonder if my girls will ever do so?"

It was fun to her in her girlhood; it was shame to her in her mature remembrance; it was agony when she saw it possible to her own children.

What a Young Woman Ought to Know

True fun is fun in anticipation, fun in realization, fun in retrospection, and fun in seeing it repeated by succeeding generations. If it fails to be fun in any of these instances, it fails to be genuine.

I like to see young people full of vivacity. I like to hear their merry laughter, to witness their innocent pranks; but I do not like to see them laughing at the sufferings of others, or amusing themselves with dangers of any kind. Above all, I regret to see them playing with the fire of physical passion.

Many a girl who to-day is lost to virtue had no idea that she was starting on this downward road. She was only having a good time. She was pretty, attractive, and admired. Young men flattered her with words, and when they held her hand, or put their arm around her, she took it as another compliment to her charms. She did not see that it was only selfishness, only a desire to feel the thrills of physical pleasure which this contact with her person aroused. She would have felt humiliated had she recognized this fact, and it seems to me that girls should understand the feelings that prompt young men to take personal familiarities.

The young man might deny the fact to the girl, but he understands it well enough as a fact, and he loses a measure of respect for her because she is willing to permit his advances. The girl no doubt imagines that these are sweet little secrets between herself and the young man, when perhaps he is discussing her openly with his young men friends. I have even heard such discussions on railway trains, carried on in no very low tones, between young men, well dressed and with all the outward appearances of gentlemen, and I have wondered how Jennie and Sadie and Clara and Nellie, whose names I heard openly mentioned, would have felt to have heard themselves described as "a nice, soft little thing to hug," or "she knows how to kiss."

Do you imagine these young men would have thus spoken had they truly respected the girls? They might say "They are nice girls," but would they say, in their deeper consciousness, "They are true, self-respecting, womanly girls, and I honor them?"

"But what is a girl to do?" asks one. "If she is prudish she won't get any attention. She has to allow a certain innocent freedom, or young men won't go with her."

Do you really believe that, dear girl? Let me tell you what young men have said to me. Said one, "O, we have to be familiar with the girls. They all expect it, and would be offended if we were just friendly and manifested no familiarities." Do you suppose girls ever thought of the possibility of the young men saying that? When they are pleading for permission to be familiar they do sometimes say, "Why, all the girls allow it," but they also add, "so there can be no harm;" while among themselves they are laughing at the credulity of the girls, or accusing them of making it necessary for the young men to take "innocent" liberties in order to have the good will of the girls.

A young man may assure you most emphatically that he respects you none the less, although you allow him to hold your hand or kiss you at parting, but he knows it is not true, and he will admit it to others rather than to the girl herself. Truthful young men say, "Of course, we have the most respect for the girls who keep us at a distance." "But they won't pay us attention," say the girls. "Is that so?" I asked of a young man. "Are you more earnest in pursuit of the girl who courts approaches, or the girl who holds you at bay?" "Why!" responded he, with emphasis, "the girls ought to know that a boy wants most that which is hardest to get; but we are actually obliged to treat the girls with familiarity or they won't go with us." And this young man seemed really surprised when I assured him that girls supposed they were obliged to accept caresses in order to have the attention of young men. Then this same young man spoke of something that I know to be too often true. He said, "It is strange, if the girls don't want these things, that they act as they do, for they actually invite familiarity. In fact, many times I would have been glad to be respectfully friendly, but the girls did not seem satisfied, and by many little ways and manners they indicated that they were ready to be caressed. I think they mean to be good girls, but they put an awful lot of temptation in a fellow's way."

No doubt these girls did not realize what they were doing, but I believe every young woman should have so clear an understanding of human nature as to know that she is playing with a dangerous fire when she allows caresses and unbecoming familiarity. She ought to know that, while she may hold herself above criminal deeds, if she permits fondlings and caresses she may be directly responsible for arousing a passion in the young man that may lead him to go out from her presence and seek the company of dissolute women, and thus lose his honor and purity because a girl who called herself virtuous tempted him. Is she in truth more honorable than the outcast woman? She has allowed familiarities in the matter of embraces and kisses, and she may not know what thoughts have been inspired in the mind of the young man by her unguarded conduct. She may feel indignant at the suggestion, because she has meant no harm, but in reality she should blush that her own familiar conduct has given him a tacit right to think of her with even greater freedom.

Girls have a wonderful responsibility in regard even to the moral conduct of young men, and the self-respecting girl will guard herself not only from the contamination of touch, but from an undue freedom of thought.

Do you say she cannot govern the thoughts of men? I reply, she can to a great extent. By a dress that exposes her person to public gaze, or even more seductively hides it under a film of suggestive lace, she has given a direction to the thoughts of those who look at her. She has declared that their eyes may touch her, that their thoughts may be occupied with an inventory of her physical charms. She has openly announced that she is willing to be appraised by eyes of men as a beautiful animal. What wonder if their thoughts go further than her public declaration, and that they may freely surmise the charms that still remain hidden?

When a girl, by putting herself into graceful attitudes in tempting nearness to a young man, casts coquettish glances, she has done that which will give a turn to the thought which may prove provocative of deeds.

"I am afraid of that girl," said a young man who desired to live purely. "May be she does not mean it, but her poses and glances make it almost impossible for me to keep my hands off of her. I am obliged to leave her for fear that I shall kiss her when she looks so mischievously alluring."

The girl, perhaps, would have been flattered by the kiss and indignant at further liberties, yet would have felt no compunctions had her victim been inflamed by a passion that he lacked the power to control, prompting him to seek some other girl to be his prey.

You think men should have self-control. So they should. We will not lessen the blame of the young man, but the girl who puts the temptation in his way, even if she did not herself yield to it, is not guiltless.

The conduct of a pure woman should be the safeguard and not the destruction of a man, and she can be his protector, even as he is hers. I heard an eminent woman say that woman was man's moral protector, and man woman's physical protector, and I said that is only half true. Man is also woman's moral protector, and woman is also man's physical protector. She is acknowledged to be his physical tempter. If she knows her power she can, by her wise, modest, womanly demeanor, make it impossible for him to feel an impure impulse in her presence. Ruskin says:

"You cannot think that the buckling on of the knight's armor by his lady's hand was a mere caprice of romantic fashion. It is the type of an eternal truth—that the soul's armor is never well set to the heart unless a woman's hand has braced it; and it is only when she braces it loosely that the honor of manhood fails. Know you not those lovely lines—I would they were learned by all youthful ladies of England—

> "'Ah wasteful woman! she who may
> On her sweet self set her own price,
> Knowing he cannot choose but pay—
> How has she cheapen'd Paradise!
> How given for nought her priceless gift,
> How spoiled the bread and spill'd the wine,
> Which, spent with due, respective thrift,
> Had made brutes men, and men divine!'"

CHAPTER XXI.

FRIENDSHIP BETWEEN BOYS AND GIRLS.

You might like to know, dear reader, if I do not believe in some intermediate relation between that of the comrade and the lover—a more intimate relation than the one and less intimate than the other. You ask, Cannot a young man and a young woman be real, true friends?

Let us talk a little about friendship and what it implies. I should define a friend as one who believes in me, who expects much of me, who encourages me to do the best that is in me, who will tell me of my faults, who recognizes my virtues, who trusts in my honor.

You are willing to accept that definition, and you think it possible to be all that to each other without being lovers. I believe it, too, but I would like to make some further statements before we have the discussion of this question.

I believe that a girl's first and best friends are her parents; her wisest *confidante*, her mother. To these she may speak unreservedly of herself. With these she may freely talk over family matters. In a friendship with some outside the family it would be unwise to discuss family matters. It might be an unkindness to other members of the family, and in case of a break in the friendship the family secrets might be betrayed, and to the detriment of the trusting friend. I once read of such an affair, where one girl had confided to another certain matters that reflected on the honor of her family, and when the friendship was broken the secret was betrayed, to the public shame of the girl who had been unwise in her confidences.

True honor would forbid the betrayal of a confidence even after the rupture of a friendship; but all persons have not the highest ideal of honor. If the girl is not discreet in her revelation of herself, and her mother is her only *confidante*, it will not be so serious a matter, for the mother will never be tempted to reveal to others anything that would bring scorn or criticism upon her child. Nowhere, in her girlish ignorance, can the girl find as sincere sympathy as in the loving mother.

"But all mothers are not sympathetic," you say. "They are often nagging, and use the confidences of the daughter to make her uncomfortable." Well, if this be so, you, at least, can learn the lesson, and by your habits of thought fit yourself to be the wise, loving, companionable, sympathetic *confidante* of your daughter, for you will be anxious that she should have no friend so close as yourself.

However, I believe that mothers should recognize the individuality of their daughters, and win, rather than command, confidence. It is difficult for us, as mothers, to realize that our daughter is just as much a separate individual as is our neighbor's daughter, and that we have no right to thrust ourselves upon her, no right to demand that she shall love us. We have the right to sympathize, to counsel, to direct her conduct so long as she remains in our personal care, but we should remember that she must be responsible, that she is a soul and must live her own life, learn her own lessons, suffer her own experiences. Our deepest love can only enable us to help her to choose wisely, to think truly, to act judiciously. So I would have the friendship of mother and daughter something very deep and true—something more than a petting and caressing, an indulging or humoring.

I would be inclined to have less outward demonstration and more inner tenderness. I believe that very often outward impression comes largely to take the place of true affection. I see girls who kiss and fondle their mothers, who never open to them their heart's deepest secrets. Fewer kisses and more confidence would satisfy more thoroughly the mother's heart. I believe that, even in the family, a kiss should not become a conventionality. It should have a meaning. I would rather that my daughter should kiss me once a week, with a spontaneous desire thus to express her love, than that, from custom, she should kiss me morning, noon, and night.

There are sanitary reasons against kissing, such as transmission of germs of disease; but aside from this, there are affectional reasons why kisses should be few, and these few spontaneous rather than required.

What a Young Woman Ought to Know

We ought never to force our kisses upon children; but, recognizing their individuality, leave them free to proffer or to refuse.

Next to the friendship of parents should come that of brother and sister. We almost think it a wonder when members of the same family seem really to love each other, and yet family ties should be the strongest in the world. Why should there not be the sweetest intimacy between two sisters, whose lives and interests are so closely united? Why should not the bond between mother and sister be indissoluble?

A young man and woman, children of the same parents, brought up in the same home, ought to be the best of friends. Their friendship is without the danger of misunderstanding. It can be free from the slight feeling of envy or jealousy that might arise between sisters. It would seem that it could be the truest comradeship possible to two young people.

A sister should be to a brother not merely some one at hand to mend his gloves or make his neckties, not simply some one to fondle and indulge, but she should be one whom he would never scold or browbeat. A brother should not be simply some one to run errands, to call on for help in emergencies, not some one to tease when the spirit of mischief prompts, or to scold when things have gone wrong.

I would have the love of these two manifest itself in all true helpfulness, but in a way that would draw out the noblest self-reliance in each. It should manifest itself in courteous words, in helpful deeds, in glances of the eye, in tones of the voice, in heartfelt sympathies that stimulate to nobler deeds, in every way that strengthens and uplifts; and if caresses are few, they will not be missed in the wealth of that truer manifestation which makes the recipient feel his nobility and worth.

A young lady once asked me if I believed in young people who were not related treating each other as brother and sister, and I replied that would depend on how the brother and sister treated each other. I have seen girls treat brothers in ways that other young men would not enjoy—finding fault, nagging, and snubbing generally. I have seen young men browbeat their sisters, tease them, and be continually unkind. I presume, if such a young man should propose to be a brother to a girl, he would not purpose to treat her in this way. Young people sometimes like to try to deceive themselves, and they fancy that the subterfuge of calling each other brother and sister will be a warrant for the parting kiss or the tender endearment that they enjoy, but which they feel proprieties will not allow. The subterfuge is too transparent. It deceives no one, and it does not make right that which, without it, would be improper.

Platonic friendships—that is, friendships between men and women without the element of physical love—are rare; rarer, indeed, than they should be. They are difficult to maintain because of the temptation to begin in the indulgences of personal familiarities, which tend to lead the friendship over into debatable ground. Men and women ought to be grand, true friends, inciting each other to the noblest achievements, but it never can be through sentimentality.

A girl may think she is sisterly when she listens to the young man's cry for sympathy in some trouble, and she holds his hand and smoothes his hair and comforts him after this tender fashion, and he may go away feeling comforted, even as a baby might be quieted by petting; but his moral fiber has not been strengthened; he has not been made to feel stronger to do and dare.

Supposing she had listened with interest to his story, and then, without laying her hands upon him, she had said, "You are a man, a prince, the son of a King. You are strong to bear, brave to do. Obstacles surmounted give broader outlooks. Burdens bravely borne bring strength. I believe in you;" and then, with a strong, firm—I had almost said manly—grasp of the hand, she had sent him away, he would go feeling stronger, braver, more self-reliant, stimulated, encouraged, not merely soothed and quieted. In this fashion a girl may treat a young man as a brother. She may tell him his faults in all kindness. She may listen to his dreams, ambitions, aspirations, and encourage with approval, incite by gentle sarcasm, or enliven by kindly sportiveness; but her person is her own, and he should be made to feel that beyond these bounds he may not pass. Such friendship may endure vicissitude, or separation, and be through life a source of truest inspiration. To be such a friend to a noble man is a worthy ambition. It would prove the possession of more qualities of womanliness than merely to win his passionate love.

When the world comes to accept the highest ideals of life and believes that all relations of men and women are not of necessity founded on physical attraction, then will such friendships be more possible, and the earth can offer no more desirable future than that in which men and women, knowing each other as immortal intelligences, shall leave the vale of unsafe sentimentality and sensuous poison to dwell on heights of noble companionship.

CHAPTER XXII.

FRIENDSHIP BETWEEN GIRLS.

You think, perhaps, that I can find no fault with the friendship of girls with each other, that that certainly is safe and pleasant. I have said enough for you to understand that I believe in reserve even in girl friendships. Girls are apt at certain periods of their lives to be rather gushing creatures. They form most sentimental attachments for each other. They go about with their arms around each other, they loll against each other, and sit with clasped hands by the hour. They fondle and kiss until beholders are fairly nauseated, and in a few weeks, perhaps, they do not speak as they pass each other, and their caresses are lavished on others. Such friendships are not only silly, they are even dangerous. They are a weakening of moral fiber, a waste of mawkish sentimentality. They may be even worse. Such friendship may degenerate even into a species of self-abuse that is most deplorable.

When girls are so sentimentally fond of each other that they are like silly lovers when together, and weep over each other's absence in uncontrollable agony, the conditions are serious enough for the consultation of a physician. It is an abnormal state of affairs, and if probed thoroughly might be found to be a sort of perversion, a sex mania, needing immediate and perhaps severe measures.

I wish the friendships of girls were less sentimental, were more manly. Two young men who are friends do not lop on each other, and kiss and gush. They trust each other, they talk freely together, they would stand by each other in any trouble or emergency, but their expressions of endearment are not more than the cordial handgrasp and the unsentimental appellation, "Dear old chap."

I admire these friendships in young men. They seem to mean so much, and yet to exact so little. They believe in each other's love, but do not demand to be told of it every minute.

It is the highest type of friendship that can believe in the friend under all circumstances. I have a friend from whom I may not hear once a year, yet I know just where she stands in her relation to me, and I would have no fear of finding her cold or unresponsive should I at any time call on her for a friendly service. I may never see her, or even hear from her again in life, and we may live long years yet on the earth, but I would as soon think of doubting the return of tomorrow's sun as to doubt her love. There is no need of words, of caresses, even of deeds. We are both busy women. Our daily cares absorb us, yet we know that we are friends, and in the great hereafter we hope to find a place where we may pause and look into each other's faces and enjoy an interchange of thought. But now other interests than self-seeking claim us. We work on, cheered by the thought that time cannot alienate us, for true love is eternal.

The charm of a true friendship is that it does not make demands. I had a school friend who thought that because she was my friend I must tell her all my affairs. She was offended if I received a letter that I did not read to her, or if I went out to spend the evening without first informing her. Her friendship became a tax because it demanded so much. And, after all, was it true friendship? Was it not love of self, rather than of me? People sometimes imagine that, because they crave love, they are affectionate and unselfish. Is it true? It is rather natural to want to be loved, but it is selfish, and the feeling indulged in to any extent is weakening. To want to be loved means usually to want some one to be a protector, a giver of pleasure, a supplier of wants. To desire to love is nobler, for to love is to give. God so loved the world that he gave. Christ loved us and gave—gave Himself for us. To love truly, grandly, nobly, is to grow strong through giving. Not giving that which we should not give, not unwisely giving of time that belongs to our own best good, not giving of strength that should be dedicated to some better purpose, not a yielding of principle, nor purity, nor honor, but the true giving of that which enriches both giver and recipient, which ennobles, uplifts, encourages and strengthens, and leaves no sorrow in its wake. The truest giving is sometimes a refusal to yield to demands that are unworthy. Love wisely, my daughter, and you will give wisely.

CHAPTER XXIII.

EXERCISES.

As many girls are affected by spinal curvature, round shoulders, weak back or ankles, prolapsed stomach, bowels, or pelvic organs, constipation and poor general circulation, it seems well to give a few exercises that shall be corrective of these defects, premising that each exercise should be begun gradually and easily, increasing frequency and force, as strength is gained, say five times a day the first week, eight times a day the second week, and so on.

Never exercise in tight clothing or in a corset, and do not *exercise to exhaustion*.

To Overcome Slight Lateral Curvature.

1. If it is the right shoulder that is depressed, place the hands on hips or behind neck, and bend slowly to the left.

Reverse this movement if the left is the lower shoulder.

2. With arms raised above the head, bend the body slowly forward and try to touch the floor without bending the knees, then rise slowly to an erect position.

To Overcome Round Shoulders.

Do not fold the arms in front.

Any motion that brings hands together behind the back is good.

Draw the elbows quickly backward.

Carry a weight in each hand, holding the weight behind you and out from the body.

Hold the body in the correct attitude (see page 132), head balanced on spine, chest elevated, posterior part of body thrown out, weight on balls of feet, not on heels.

Exercises that strengthen the waist muscles will help to maintain the erect position, and so tend to overcome round shoulders.

To Strengthen Weak Back.

1. Hold a light weight in each hand. Place the weights on the floor in front of you. Stand with feet eight inches apart, and take three slow, deep breaths. Stoop over and take the weights in the hands and gradually straighten up till the hands hang easily at the sides. Bend slowly forward, and again place the weights on the floor. Repeat five times.

2. Clasp the hands back of the neck and bend slowly forward until the head is on a level with the waist. Count ten, then straighten up to erect position. Repeat.

3. Bend the body backward, forward and sidewise at the waist.

4. Put your right arm over your head till it touches your left ear. Hold the chin high. Breathe slowly and deeply while you walk around the room. Repeat with other arm. Increase the length of your walk gradually.

5. Playing tennis is good exercise for the sides of the waist.

6. Carry a weight first on one shoulder, then on the other.

7. Run on the toes.

8. Hop on one foot.

To Strengthen and Develop the Chest.

1. Maintain an erect attitude.

2. Raise and lower the arm, forward, upward, backward, without bending the elbows.

3. Lie on the floor, stretch the arms over the head till the hands touch the floor. Take a deep breath and hold it; now bring the arms over the head as high as you can reach, and do not bend the elbows. Rest and repeat three times.

4. Hold chin as high as possible. Raise the arms at the side as high as you can. Breathe deeply and hold the air in the lungs. Now, without letting any air out and without bending the elbows, bring your hands down steadily to your sides. Repeat. Keep chin well up.

To Strengthen Abdominal Muscles.

1. Stand with chin high.

2. Breathe slowly and deeply.

3. Raise the right knee till the right foot is about twelve inches from the floor.

4. Give a little spring with the left foot, raise it swiftly from the floor, and at the same time put the right toe and sole (not heel) to the floor.

5. Spring on right foot and put left down. Repeat five times.

6. Fold arms behind. Hold chin up. Breathe slowly and very deeply. Do not bend the knees. Hold your left foot far out in front of you while you count five.

7. Lower it and raise right foot in same way. Repeat four times. Keep the shoulders well back and down while doing this exercise. Point the toes down and out.

8. Lie on your back. Keep feet down and rise to a sitting position. Drop slowly back, and repeat three times.

9. Run, lifting your feet high, like a spirited horse.

10. Stand with chin high, arms akimbo. Breathe slowly and deeply. Advance left foot eight inches in front of right. Lean head slowly as far back as possible. Hold it while you count five. Straighten, and repeat five times.

11. Place the hands on the wall in front of you as high as you can reach and about two feet apart, with the elbows straight. Have chin up till you face the ceiling, and keep it so. Take a very deep breath and hold it. Now bend your elbows and let the body go slowly forward till the chest touches the wall, keeping the body and legs

stiff all the time. Push back till straight again. Do not take heels off the floor, nor hands off the wall, nor eyes off the ceiling right overhead. Repeat five times.

12. Lie on the floor, stretch the arms over the head till the hands touch the floor. Clinch the fists. Take a deep breath and hold it. Now raise the arms slowly, keeping the fists clinched, and bring them down at the sides, raising the head from the floor at same time. Raise the arms and stretch them on the floor over the head at same time, letting the head sink back to the floor, and breathe out slowly.

To Facilitate the Return of Displaced Organs to Their Normal Position.

1. Lie on your back upon a smooth, hard surface. Draw the feet up as close to the body as possible. Now lift the lower part of the body until it is wholly supported by the feet and shoulders. Hold it in this position as long as possible without fatigue. Lower slowly to original position. Rest a few minutes. Repeat. Continue for twenty or thirty minutes, according to strength.

2. Lie with face downward. Raise the hips as high as possible, supporting the body on the toes and elbows.

3. Slip from the bed head first and face downwards until the head rests on the floor and the legs and feet remain upon the bed. Let the arms to the elbows rest on the floor. When weary of this attitude slip to the floor, turn on the back, and apply the bandage.

CHAPTER XXIV.

RECREATIONS.

Walking.

It is well to bear constantly in mind that all exercise, even walking on level ground, is objectionable in clothing that compresses the body; and as exercise is the law of the development of muscle, the only safe thing to do is so to dress that every muscle has free and unrestrained motion. Walking to be beneficial should be out of doors, with some pleasant motive, and taken with some degree of energy. The length of the walk should be proportional to the strength of the girl—short at first, and increasing as strength increases. The erect attitude should be maintained, and the walking not prolonged to exhaustion.

Walking slowly home from school, laden with books and intent on conversation with others, will not fulfill the demands of walking for exercise. It makes no demand on breathing power, does not develop depth of chest or strength of limb.

Running.

This is an admirable exercise if the dress be suitable. Long skirts are an impediment. Running on the toes develops the calf of the leg.

The swift motion causes deep breathing, which expands the chest. If violent or long-continued, it may make too urgent a demand on the heart and lungs, and so be detrimental. The counsel of a physician is safest for those whose heart and lungs are weak.

Riding.

Horseback riding is a vigorous exercise, which would be especially beneficial were it not for the cramped position women are forced by custom to assume. It cannot be recommended to those who have a tendency to lateral curvature of the spine or weak back, or prolapsed internal organs. Such girls should by proper care be put into a better physical condition before attempting to ride. Harvey advises learning to ride on either side of the horse, so as to bring opposite sets of muscles into play, and counteract the curvature which physicians who have the opportunity to observe say is produced by riding. That being true, why not adopt the sensible fashion of riding on both sides of the horse at once, as men do? I saw a young lady so mounted the other day, and the sight was far more agreeable than the twisted attitude compelled by the side-saddle. Medical men also assert that riding tends to produce round shoulders, and as the greatest muscular strain comes on the back, it is not helpful to weak backs.

Skating.

Skating is a fine exercise. It quickens the circulation and the respiration, aids digestion, exercises a great number of muscles, both of limbs and trunk of body, strengthens the ankles, and incidentally the nerves. Evils are to be found in wrong habits of dressing, the tendency to overdo through the fascination of the sport, the danger of taking cold by carelessly sitting down to rest when heated, or driving home after being warmed up by the severe exertion. A girl of good judgment, properly clothed, ought to be benefited by this charming out-door sport.

It should be begun very gradually at the opening of the skating season, and not undertaken if the internal organs are prolapsed.

Rowing.

Rowing is an exercise that develops the upper back and back of shoulders, and therefore needs to be counteracted by exercise that calls into play the muscles of the front of the chest.

Cycling.

The dangers of cycling arise principally from lack of judgment. The temptation to overdo is very great, and injury is done in attempts to ride longer, farther and faster than the strength will safely allow. The whole dress should be so arranged as to give perfect freedom of movement, the skirt short enough to clear the dangerous part of the mechanism, the saddle adjusted to the individual both in its make and height, and the girl be taught to sit properly and to adjust her weight so that the pressure will not be undue upon the perineum.

Rectal and other local irritations are produced by the pressure of the whole weight resting on the saddle.

The position should not be absolutely erect, but leaning *slightly* forward, so as to allow the weight to be distributed between the handle-bars, the pedal, and the saddle. This slightly inclined attitude also maintains the proper and harmonious relation of the internal organs, so that the bowels do not crowd down on the pelvic organs.

If the girl is taught to sit on the machine properly, to distribute her weight, to sit on the large gluteal muscles, and not on the perineum, to use judgment in the amount of exercise taken at a time, there is no reason why a girl in a normal condition of health should not be benefited.

There may be particular reasons why some girls should not undertake to ride, and these can be determined by the physician.

Tennis.

This is a game that demands great activity, consequently there is especial need of entire freedom of movement. All constrictions of clothing are especially injurious.

It is claimed by some that, being essentially a one-sided exercise, there is a possibility, if unwisely indulged in, that it may produce injurious results, especially to the spine.

Swimming.

Swimming is not only a valuable exercise, but it really conduces to the safety of life in these days of constant boat travel, and there are no adequate reasons why girls should not learn. The younger they begin, the more readily will they become expert. It is not wise to indulge in this exercise while menstruating, nor immediately after eating.

Skipping.

There is some prejudice against this form of exercise from the fact that it can be overdone, and also from the popular idea that it is injurious to girls to jump.

If they are properly dressed, and their muscles are gradually developed, and they use good common sense as to amount, there are practically no dangers in skipping. It is admirably adapted to strengthen a great variety of muscles, as those of the legs, back, abdomen, and neck. It strengthens the knees and the arches of the feet, thereby tending to overcome flat foot. It strengthens weak backs, increases circulation and respiration and promotes digestion, and, if practised out of doors, is one of the most perfect forms of exercise. Of course the judgment dictates that when the pelvic organs are heavy with the menstrual congestion it would not be advisable.

Dancing.

Dancing, in itself considered, is a pleasant and beneficial exercise. It develops grace and muscular strength, increases circulation and respiration, and is cheering because of rhythm. One wishes that it could be unqualifiedly commended. But when we take into account the late hours, the heated rooms, the promiscuous company, the late unwholesome suppers, the improper dress, the dangers of taking cold, the immodest freedom of the round dance, and the not infrequent evils resulting therefrom, it would seem unwise to commend an exercise so surrounded by objectionable concomitants. It is observed that young church members who become interested in the dance soon lose all their interest in church work.

If dancing could be conducted in the daytime, out of doors, among well-known home friends and companions, in proper dress, and with *no round dances,* there would be much to commend, and little to condemn.

Card-playing.

I can find little to say in favor of this form of amusement. It contains no exercise for the body. It continues the cramped attitudes to which most people are condemned during the day.

It certainly contributes nothing to the higher forms of enjoyment. It stimulates emulations, which St. Paul enumerates among things to be avoided; it is the accompaniment of gambling and low society; and, while we must admit that a pack of cards in itself is not evil, yet it can be and often is made most detrimental to the best interests of morality and righteousness.

The young woman who respects her own intellectual and moral powers will see little charm in manipulating cards in a way to gain a momentary success over another and perhaps arousing unkind feelings, it may be even passions, that may culminate in bloodshed.

Theatre-going.

It is natural that we should enjoy pictorial representation of human life with living actors and audible words; and, understanding this, many good people have had the hope that the stage might be purified and made a teacher of morals. Certainly valuable lessons of life might be most strongly presented in this concrete form, and thus appeal with wonderful power to the young and inexperienced. But that it might be so used does not insure that it will be, and observation shows us that it is not.

The modern play concerns itself principally with a delineation of those phases of life which we condemn when they become reality, and the teaching power of the stage becomes a lesson in wrongdoing which to the young and inexperienced is potent in its suggestiveness.

The costumes of actresses are often immodest, and many of these women are immoral in character. It would not be just to condemn all actors with the sweeping assertion of immorality, but all will admit that the temptations are great, and that great moral force is needed to resist the influences that lead towards wrong.

That many of our great actors will not permit their children to become actors, or, in some cases, even to enter the theatre as a witness of its performances, speaks strongly on the matter.

In the consideration of this subject the girl may safely decide that she will not be a permanent loser if she is not a frequenter of the theatre. It is safer to keep the mind pure and untainted from all pictures of sin, more especially if they are made attractive by the glamour of jewels and silken attire, of music, dancing, and lifelike portrayal.

PART III.
LOVE; HEREDITY; ENGAGEMENTS.

CHAPTER XXV.

LOVE.

In our study we have first learned of general and then of special physiology, so, in continuing the same study in mental and moral fields, we first learn of the general and then of our special relation to others. We cultivate body, mind and spirit because it is our duty to develop ourselves for our own interests; but it is also our duty to cultivate all our powers because of our responsibility in regard to others. This responsibility I will include in the one word, "love."

What is love? The idea of love occupies much of the thought of old and young, and in different persons it will have very different meanings. To one it means merely pleasurable sensations aroused by either the thought of a person, or by the actual presence of that person. To another it means an opportunity to sacrifice inclination and pleasure in order to promote the happiness or welfare of a certain person.

Much that passes in the world as love is principally love of self. The man loves the woman because she satisfies his sense of beauty; her presence causes thrills and ecstasies; she contributes to his happiness and comfort. That is, he loves himself through her. The woman loves the man because he protects her, he surrounds her with luxury, his presence brings thrills and ecstasies to her. She loves herself through him. Is not this but the essence of selfishness? In another case the man loves the woman so tenderly that he cannot do enough to prove his devotion. If her welfare demands his absence, he gladly foregoes the pleasure of her society. If her comfort requires his unremitting toil, he gives his days, and even his nights, to the task of labor for her. His only anxiety is to know her wants and to supply them. He effaces himself and his wishes to serve her. He would die to secure her good. He gives, and asks nothing. Or, in the same way, the woman loves the man so that her whole thought is not what she can obtain from him, but what she can give him. True love desires only to give. Self-love strives only to secure.

Emerson says, "All the world loves a lover," and conversely we may say a true lover loves all the world. The affection kindled in the heart by one worthy individual goes out in a kindlier feeling for all the world. A poet once said that the world was brighter and all humanity dearer because he loved truly one worthy woman. He was more gentle with little children; the very beggar on the street corner seemed to be a brother in distress. Because the woman he loved had given him her heart, he wanted to give something to every one he met. This is the spirit of true love, to go out in blessings towards the beloved object, and so on towards every created thing.

I was once asked if I believed in love at first sight. How can love spring up in a minute? There may be admiration of beauty, there may be appreciation of intellectual qualities, there may be a recognition of magnetic personal attraction, but none of these is love. Love, to be worthy the name, must be a superstructure built upon a firm foundation of acquaintance with each other's true qualities. Love is not a balloon, in which two young people may go sailing among the clouds, away from all regions of every-day life. Those who try it with that idea find the cloud-world cold and uncomfortable, and not at all the rosy, gold-tinted region it looked at a distance.

Love is rather like a building with foundations set into the earth — foundations solid, firmly laid and durable. How can people love when they do not know each other? Acquaintance first, then friendship, comradeship; then, if the sentiment grows, love. But how are young people to get really acquainted? They meet under unreal conditions. They see each other in society, in Sunday dress and with Sunday manners. They doubtless do not mean to deceive each other, but there is little to draw out the real self. There is nothing to disturb or irritate, nothing to prove the honesty, the neatness, the industry, the persistence, the business ability; nothing to disclose the true ideas in matters of serious import, of health, religion, duties of husbands and wives, the government of the home; and too often the intimacy of marriage discloses many personal peculiarities of temper, habits and manners that, if seen in time, would have prevented marriage.

The trouble does not originate with young people themselves, but with older people; but as the young people of to-day will be the older people of the future, it would be well for them to realize what the trouble is. The fact is, that in the present conditions of society the association of young people is unnatural. From earliest childhood boys and girls are taught to think of each other only in sentimental ways. The little boys and girls in school are playing at "lovering," and their conversation is often more about beaus and sweethearts than about the plays of childhood, which alone should occupy their thoughts. You remember that little miss of ten who asked you, when you were sixteen, who was your beau. You recall her look of surprise when you replied that you had none, and her exclamation, "Have no beau! Why, how do you get along without one?" What made such a mere child imagine a beau to be an essential agent of a girl's life? Because she had been taught by the jests and suggestions of her elders that every boy was a possible lover, and, young as she was, that thought was woven into her very life. It is pitiable to see how early the mind of the child is tainted by sentimentality, by the unwise suggestions of older friends. I remember hearing of a child of six who was talking of getting married. Some one said, "You are too little to think of getting married," and the child replied, "Why, I have thought of it since I was two years old." And doubtless she had, because it had been continually impressed on her mind by the conversation of parents and friends, and the direction they had given her thought in regard to her relation to everything masculine.

Parents are often very unwilling to teach their daughters the facts of sex, and yet quite willing to emphasize the consciousness of sex by intimating the possibility of flirtations, love affairs, etc. And this false, pernicious idea of the relation of men and women is too often called love. The central idea of romances is this passionate attraction of the sexes. The plot gathers in intensity around the lovers, and culminates in their marriage, after which life is presumed to move on without a jar, and silly girls and impulsive boys imagine that the sweet pain that accompanies the touch of hands or the glance of the eyes is love, and is a sufficient guarantee for the forming of a life partnership.

Let us face this question fairly. What is love? Of what is it made? Can you judge with any certainty of its lasting qualities? How can you know the true from the false?

Unfortunately we have but the one word, "love," to designate many phases of kindly regard. The mother loves her child, the child loves the mother, yet love differs much in these two instances. The one is protecting, anxious, self-sacrificing, unstinted care, unqualified devotion; the other is sweet dependence, unquestioning acceptance, asking all and giving little. The love of brother and sister differs from that of brother for brother, or sister for sister. The love of man for woman differs from all other emotions of love. It contains elements not found in other forms. It may have the same quality of giving or accepting, of protecting or yielding, but with all this there is an added quality that is not found in any other relation of life, a quality that rises to the intensity of a passion, and which, if thwarted or distorted, may become murderous or lead to insanity.

This overwhelming, domineering sway of feeling inheres in the fact of sex. It is the expression of the whole nature, through the physical; it is the vital creative force endeavoring to reach a tangible result. Holy in its inception, it can be degraded to the vilest uses. Forming the distinctive feature of love between the sexes, it is too often imagined to be the all, and a strong physical attraction without the basic friendship, which can only come through acquaintance, is not infrequently supposed to be worthy of the name of love, and found, alas! to be the most unsubstantial of chimeras.

Love, to be worthy of the name, must rest, not on the fact of admiration for beauty, not on the physical attraction manifested in sweet electric thrills. Love should include intellectual congeniality and spiritual sympathy, as well as physical attraction. Lacking any one of these three ingredients, the interest of two people in each other should not be called love.

In order that it may be determined whether there is the true basis of love, there should be opportunity for unsentimental acquaintance. If we could free the minds of young people from the romantic idea, and allow them to associate as intelligent beings, and so form acquaintance on the basis of comradeship, we should make things safer for them.

But if the older people do not know how to secure this desirable state of affairs, the young people themselves might secure it if they understood its desirability. You, as a young woman, can have much influence in the right directions, supposing that you drop from your mind the idea of sentimental relations with young men and meet them on the ground of a friendly comradeship.

Don't indulge in *tête-à-têtes*, or in lackadaisical glances of the eye. Don't permit personal familiarities, hand pressures, or caresses. Don't simper, and put on the airs which mean, though the girl may not understand it, an effort to arouse the admiration and the physical feeling of love. Refuse to be flattered, to be played with, to be treated as a female, but insist on being treated as a woman with intelligence, with a capacity to understand reasonable things. Manifest an interest in the movements of the world, of politics, literature, art, religion, athletics. Talk of the things that interest the young man as a citizen of the world, and not merely of those things which appeal to him as a male. Be frank, be lively, be witty, be wise, but do not be sentimental.

When a young man calls, don't let him get the idea that you have to be secluded in a room apart from the rest of the family. You will be better able to judge of him if you see him with your brothers, if you note his manner towards your mother, if you hear him converse with your father, if you mark his conduct towards the younger children. He will talk sense, if he can, when he meets your family, while in a *tête-à-tête* conversation with yourself he may be able to hide his lack of wisdom under the glamour of sweet nothings and soft nonsense.

Then be yourself when he comes. Let him see you in your home life, at your domestic duties, sewing, helping mother, reading to father, caring for the little ones. Be an honest, free-hearted, companionable girl, and put sentimentality out of mind. You can have many such friends, and by and by, out of these you will probably find one whom you admire more and more as time goes on. You hear his sentiments always expressed in favor of truth and probity. You come to know something of his business principles, you see his courtesy to old and young, you learn of his home, his family, his social position, and out of this intimate knowledge there springs the attachment, blended with deep respect, which assures you that he is worthy of your heart and hand, and indeed of your whole life.

Little by little the comradeship has grown more intimate. You have not been sentimental. You have treated each other with respect, you have maintained your self-respect, you have held a tight rein over your fancies and emotions, but now you are convinced that you may allow them to have sway. You begin to acknowledge to yourself that you love.

And he, too, begins to manifest a deeper interest in you. You see this with a certain pride in the fact that he is not self-deceived He knows you, has seen you in your daily life, has sounded the depth of your intellect, knows of your religious beliefs, and in all he has found you coming up to his ideals. His eye meets yours with a new tenderness in its glance that touches you, because you know it is not an earthly fire of passion that glows therein. It is you, the real, immortal you, that he seeks; not merely the pleasures of sense through you; and feeling the response in your own heart, your glance kindles with the same divine fire, and your true selves have spoken to each other. You have gradually grown into the knowledge of love. You have not fallen in love. And yet there have been no words, and in maiden shyness you await his speech. Your womanly reserve has won his respect, and he makes no attempts to win privileges of endearments before he confesses his love, but frankly and manfully pleads his suit and wins.

Oh, my dear child, this has been no matter for jesting; it has been serious, and we who have watched this dawning love have realized that the great drama of life, so full of tragic possibilities, is being here enacted. We do not laugh, nor jest, but with the tenderest prayers we welcome you into the possibilities of God's divinest gift of human love.

CHAPTER XXVI.

RESPONSIBILITY IN MARRIAGE.

You are beginning to feel a peculiar interest in one young man more than in any other. You think of him in his absence; you welcome his coming; his eyes seem to caress you; the clasp of his hand thrills you; you begin to think that you have passed from the domain of friendship into that of love.

Before you really make that admission, let us "reason together." Let us take a fair look at matters, and see whether it is wiser to pass the border line, or to remain only friends. Who is this young man? You tell me his name, but that means nothing. Who is he? What is he in himself? What are his talents, capacities, habits, inherited tendencies? Who is his father, his mother? What is their worth? I do not mean in money, but in themselves? What ancestral diseases or defects may he transmit to his posterity, which will be your posterity if he becomes your husband? Are the family tendencies such that you would be willing to see them repeated in your children?

There is no indelicacy in asking yourself these questions, nor in making the investigations which will enable you to answer them satisfactorily. The woman who marries, marries not only *into* her husband's family, she also marries his family; she is to become one of it, to live with it in closer and closer companionship as her children, bearing the family temperament, disposition and tendencies, gather one by one around her hearth.

Is the family one of the type that she will desire to associate with intimately all the days of her life? You may feel that it does not matter if you do not love your husband's mother, or admire his sisters; no matter if you do not have respect for his father, you will live so far away from them that it will not be oftener than once in several years that you will be obliged to meet them. It might even happen that you would never see them, and yet it be a very serious matter that they were not respectable or lovable people, for they constitute one-half of the ancestry of your children. Their most undesirable characteristics may, perchance, be the endowment of your sons and daughters, and your heart ache, or even break, over the habits, or, it may be, criminality, which may disgrace your home through the paternal inheritance that you chose for them. Viewed in this light, marriage becomes a most serious matter. It is unfortunate that girls generally have the idea that it is not modest to think of marriage further than the ceremony. Of the responsibilities and duties they are not only ignorant, but think it ladylike to remain uninformed until experience teaches them, and that teaching is often accompanied by heart-breaking sorrow. If you should make inquiry you would discover that a large proportion of mothers have buried their firstborn children, and should you ask them why, they would in all probability say, almost without exception, that it was because they did not know how to give them a dower of health, or how to care for their physical needs.

Again, investigation would show you that children go astray, become wild, dissipated, or even criminal, because parents have not known how to train them, how to keep their confidence, how wisely to guide them in ways of righteousness.

We all believe it very important that mothers should know how to direct and govern their children, and yet we do not train the future mothers for this important office. We teach girls how to sew or cook, how to embroider and play the piano. We do not expect them to know, without instruction, how to mingle the ingredients for a cake or pudding, but we imagine that they will know by intuition how to secure the best results in the mingling of heterogeneous compounds in the formation of the characteristics of a human being.

When we speak of the mother's privilege, we think of the actual mother, whose privilege is to care for and guide her real children. But the mother's privilege in fact begins in her own childhood, when by her habits of life and thought she is deciding her own character, and at the same time creating, in great degree, the talents and tendencies of her possible children. It is her privilege to secure a measure of physical vigor for her descendants by her care of her own health in her very girlhood. She can endow them with mental power by not frittering away her own powers of mind in foolish reading or careless methods of study. By her own self-respecting conduct she helps to give them the reverence for self which will insure their acting wisely. All this is the mother's privilege; and still one more great privilege is hers, and that is to choose one-half the ancestry of her descendants. She cannot choose their ancestry that comes to them through herself; that is a fixed fact. Her parents must of necessity be her children's grandparents. Her family characteristics are also their inheritance. The only thing she can do in regard to their inheritance through her is to modify the objectionable traits, and to cultivate the good traits herself, so that family faults may in her be weakened and the probability of transmission lessened, and the family virtues be strengthened and their probable transmission intensified. But she has the power to decide what shall be the paternal ancestry of her household; and if she is duly impressed with the responsibility of this power, she will not allow herself to fall in love and marry a man of whose family she knows nothing, or knows facts that do not promise well for posterity.

CHAPTER XXVII.

THE LAW OF HEREDITY.

I once heard of a man who on his death-bed made a singular will. He had no houses or lands to bequeath his children, but he had observed that they had inherited much from him, and so he made a formal bequest to them of that which they already possessed.

He wrote: "I bequeath to my son John my big bony frame and the slouching gait I acquired by carelessness, also my inherited tendency to consumption. To my daughter Mary I bequeath my sallow complexion and torpid liver, which are the result of my gross living; also my melancholy disposition and tendency to look on the dark side of life. To my son Samuel I give my love for alcoholic liquors and my irritable disposition; to my daughter Jane my coarseness of thought and my unwillingness to be restrained in my desires, and also my tendency to commit suicide."

"A very strange will," said everybody, and yet it was a will that was probated long before the testator's death. That it gave perfect satisfaction I will not assert, but it was never contested and paid no fees to lawyers.

Just such wills are being made daily by the lives and conduct of young people, though they are not put into writing. Some time in the future, however, they will be written into "living epistles, known and read of all men."

Other wills are being made daily that through sober, virtuous, youthful lives will bequeath to posterity dowers of health, strength, purity and power.

This being true, it seems only a part of prudent foresight to study in youth the law that governs the transmission of personal characteristics to the future "denizens of life's great city." This law is known as Heredity, and its first written record is in the first chapter of Genesis, where it is written that "Every plant and animal shall bring forth after its kind." We are so accustomed to seeing the results of this law that we give it little or no thought. We see that grass springs up each year on our lawns and meadows. We know that if we put the seeds of a certain flower in the ground, that kind of flower will always spring up, never another kind. The farmer is not anxious, after he sows wheat, for fear that the crop will be rye or barley. We expect that the young of cats will be kittens, of geese will be goslings, of men will be human children, and we are never disappointed. The law holds good under all circumstances.

We see, too, that there are certain race characteristics that maintain. The Mongolian race has peculiar high cheek-bones, sallow complexions and eyes set in bias, and we recognize the Japanese or Chinese at once, even though dressed in the garb of our country. So, too, we recognize the African or the Caucasian by certain marked characteristics. This transmission of racial traits we call race heredity.

Then each race has its own traits, physical or mental, which we recognize as national, and so speak of them. We always mention thrift as an attribute of the Teutonic nations; the Irishman we characterize as witty and pugnacious; the Frenchman as polite; the American as progressive.

Each individual has not only his human inheritance, his race inheritance and his national characteristics, but he has also an endowment of family traits.

But we are not made up of odds and ends of ancestral belongings alone. We have in ourselves something that is original, that makes us different from each other, and from all others. I have sometimes thought that we are somewhat like patchwork quilts, the parti-colored blocks being set together by some solid-colored material; or, better still, we are like "hit and miss" rag carpets, with a warp of our own individuality, filled in with a woof made of qualities and capacities of all those who have preceded us. You know, in making "hit and miss" rag carpets we take little strips and bits of various materials and all colors, and sew them together without regard to order or arrangement, and these long strips are woven back and forth in the warp until the carpet is woven, showing no set pattern, but a mingling of tints and shades that is sometimes crude and unsightly, sometimes soft and artistic.

I used, in childhood, to find great delight in seeking among the blended colors in the carpet for scraps of clothing which I recognized as having belonged to father or mother, or perhaps even to grandparents. Even now, in my maturer years, I am interested in finding in myself the physical, mental or moral characteristics of those same ancestors; and you, no doubt, can do the same, while some of your traits seem to be yours entirely, constituting individual variations upon ancestral inheritances.

Nature has been doing for centuries, unheeded, what the photographer of to-day thinks is a modern discovery, that is, making composite photographs of us all.

Through this law of inheritance have arisen the intellectual, the moral or the criminal types of humanity, and the process is continuing; the types are becoming more and more marked, or modifying influences are being brought in to change the type.

These influences are also the result of law, even though we may not be able to trace them to their cause. Knowing this, however, we begin to see that heredity is not fatality; that the power to modify the endowments of future generations is ours. To know how to employ it, we should study the law as far as we have opportunity.

This subject is a large one, and no doubt you will some day want to give it a thorough investigation. Just now, however, you will have to accept my statements. I will not make them technical, but strictly practical to you as a young woman desiring that knowledge which shall best fit you for the responsibilities of future life.

A superficial study is rather discouraging. We see with what certainty evil characteristics are transmitted, and we feel that the law is a cruel one; but if we have patience we shall find that, like all laws of God, its purpose is for the benefit of the race. Before we begin to take comfort from the law let us first learn its warnings, one of which is that all weakening of the individual, either in bodily strength, in intellectual power or moral fiber, tends to produce a like weakness in posterity. This is why I say to you that the young people of the present have in their hands the welfare of the future. Their habits to-day are moulding the possibilities of the race. Young women may feel that their individual violation of the laws of health is of no importance, but when they realize that the girls of to-day are the mothers of the future, and that the physical strength or weakness of each individual girl affects the average health of the nation, not only now, but it may be through her posterity for centuries, we can see that each girl's health is a matter of national and of racial importance.

But it is not alone in the physical organization that we can trace the law of heredity in the transmission of undesirable qualities. We find that evil traits and tendencies of mind or morals are transmissible. Galton finds that a bad temper is quite sure to be passed on from one generation to the next, and any peculiarity of disposition in either parents is quite likely to become an inheritance of the child. This fact makes our little faults seem of vastly more importance than otherwise. We can endure them in ourselves, but they strike us very unpleasantly when we are obliged to see them manifested in our children. As the poet says:

> "Little faults unheeded, which I now despise;
> For my baby took them with her hair and eyes."

It may not strike us very unpleasantly when we speak disrespectfully to our parents, but when our own children show us lack of courtesy and cheerful obedience it cuts deeply, and all the more deeply if we see in their conduct but a repetition of our own.

Of course, if these minor faults are transmissible, we will not be surprised that graver moral defects are passed on. The grandson of a thief began to steal at three years of age, and at fourteen was an expert pickpocket. The police records show the same family names recurring year after year.

These cases are so grave as to attract attention, while we overlook the fact that the smaller immoralities are as apt to be transmitted, and perhaps with increased power. I should be afraid that slight lack of strict integrity in the father might appear as actual crime in the son.

I would not omit to mention also the law of Atavism, in this discussion of heredity. This is that expression of the law in the omission of one generation in the transmission of a quality. We sometimes see the peculiarities or defects of a man or woman not manifested in their children, but reappearing in their grandchildren.

Not long ago I was in a family where both parents and all the children had dark hair but one, and she had long, bright auburn ringlets. I asked, "Where did you get your hair?"

"From my red-headed grandmother," she answered, with a laugh, indicating that the matter had been so often discussed in her hearing that she understood it quite fully.

To cover the whole scope of the law of heredity would take more time than we have to spare. You can follow out the line of thought, and make practical application of the facts and principles here laid down.

CHAPTER XXVIII.

HEREDITARY EFFECTS OF ALCOHOL, TOBACCO, ETC.

Civilized life in its progress is accompanied by certain customs and habits which are detrimental to the individual health, and therefore to national health. The dress of women is not merely an unimportant matter, to be made the subject of sneers or jests. Fashions often create deformities, and are therefore worthy of most philosophic consideration, especially when we know that the effects of these deformities may be transmitted.

The tightly-compressed waist of the girl displaces her internal organs, weakens her digestion, and deprives her children of their rightful inheritance. They are born with lessened vitality, with diminished nerve power, and are less likely to live, or, living, are more liable not only to grow up physically weak, but also lacking in mental and moral stamina. This weakness may manifest itself in immoral tendencies, or in some form of inebriety. It is now recognized that alcoholism will produce nerve degeneration, but it is not so well understood that nerve degeneration may be a factor in producing inebriates from alcohol or other poisons.

Dr. Crothers says: "Hysteria, convulsions, unreasonable anger, excitement, depression, credulity, skepticism, most unusual emotionalism and faulty reasoning, are some of the signs of nerve degeneration," and adds that this central failure of nerve and brain power is often accompanied by a resulting alcohol or drug inebriety. That is, the weak and degenerate nerves crave a stimulant, and the weak will yield to the demand, and inebriety result. If this degeneration of nerve comes from the low vitality given by the mother, because of her unhealthful habits of dress and life, is it not wise that in her early womanhood she should know of this possibility, and guard against it through her care of herself?

She ought also to understand the effect of alcohol and other poisons in producing nerve degeneration in the individual, and its probability in his posterity.

What a Young Woman Ought to Know

George McMichaels says: "The hereditary nature of the abnormal condition of which inebriety is the outward sign is not understood, even by physicians, as it should be. It is still, I regret to say, looked upon as a vice acquired by the individual, the outcome of voluntary wrongdoing. In some few cases this may be true, but in the majority of instances inquiry into the family history will reveal the presence of an inherited taint, such families usually showing a neurotic condition. No position in the social or intellectual world is, or ever has been, entirely free from the tendency towards alcoholism, and a study of the family history of the great men who have fallen victims to alcohol will show that the cause has been identical with the case among the most obscure of mankind, viz.: That a degenerated nerve condition has been inherited which renders the sufferer specially susceptible to this and allied neuroses, such as epilepsy, idiocy and suicide. The inheritance of an unstable nervous system makes the individual easily affected by what I must call 'alcoholic surroundings.' In other words, the provocation to drink which would have no influence upon an ordinary, stable nervous organization, is sufficient to turn the neurotic into a confirmed drunkard."

As a young woman you hold great power over the race in yourself, and through your influence over others, especially over young men. Your influence, wisely used, may save more than one from a drunkard's fate, and to use it wisely you should be instructed as to the real character of alcohol and its effects on the system. I have not time to tell you in minutiæ of the effects of alcohol, but I must take time to speak of the law of heredity in this respect.

Idiocy and inebriety are on the increase among civilized peoples. This startling fact should make us ask the reason.

T.D. Crothers, M.D., who is making a life study of inebriety, states that from 1870 to 1890 inebriety increased in proportion to the population over 100 per cent., and that a large proportion is the result of inebriety in one or both parents. It is a sad fact that many women, even of good social standing, are fond of alcoholic beverages. I saw a very bright, pretty young woman not long since, at a reception, refuse to take ice-cream or cake, but drink four glasses of punch, with many jests as to her fondness for the same, apparently without any glimmering of the thought that she was drinking to excess, although her flushed face and loudness of manner were proof of this to those who were witnesses. Many people have an idea that the finer drinks, such as wine and its various disguises, do not intoxicate, but in this they are mistaken. All alcoholics are intoxicating in just the degree that they contain alcohol. The exhilaration of wine is but the first step of intoxication, and that means always an accompanying lack of judgment, a lessening of the sense of propriety.

One young woman who, under ordinary circumstances, was most modest in deportment, drank at her wedding in response to the toasts to her health, and grew very jovial, until at last she danced a jig on the platform at the railway station amid the applause of her exhilarated friends, who had accompanied the young husband and wife to the train, as they started on their wedding-journey. What a sorrowful and undignified beginning to the duties of marriage!

There is no absolute safety for either man or woman except in total abstinence. The *débauché* knows the effect of wine, and uses that knowledge to lead astray the young girl who, if herself, would find no charm in his blandishments, but who, after the wine supper, has no will to resist his advances.

A young husband exacted of his bride a promise that she would never take a glass of wine except in his company, and when asked the reason, replied that he knew that no woman's judgment was to be trusted after taking one glass of wine.

Another cause of inebriety in women is found in the patent medicines advertised as a panacea for all pain, which chemical analysis shows to be largely alcoholic. Many temperance women would be horrified to know that they are taking alcohol in varying quantity, from 6 to 47 per cent., in the bitters, tonics and restorative medicines they are using, many of which are especially advertised as "purely vegetable extracts, perfectly harmless, sustaining to the nervous system," etc.

The result of inebriety of parents in inflicting injury upon offspring has not been well understood in the past, but is becoming recognized. Dr. McMichael says:

"In every form of insanity the disease is more dangerous in the mother than in the father, as far as the next generation is concerned. This is a good and sufficient reason why the daughter of drunken parents, very often attractive to some men by reason of their excitable, vivacious, neurotic manner, should be carefully avoided by young men in search of wives. The man who marries the daughter of an inebriate not only endangers his own happiness, but runs the risk of entailing upon his children an inheritance of degradation and misery.

"No woman should marry a man who, even occasionally, drinks to excess. Further, the disposition of the sons of drunken parents ought to be investigated before any girl becomes engaged to one of them. This is one instance in which long engagements are not to be condemned, for, if the man has inherited the alcoholic craving, it may become known in time, and his *fiancée* may be saved from the most terrible fate that I can think of—becoming the wife of a drunkard.

"One word more before I leave this aspect of the subject. As the majority of inebriates are sufferers from a disease which is partly the result of hereditary predisposition, it is foolish for any woman to marry a drunkard in the belief that she can reform him. If women would realize that alcoholism is a disease and not a vice, they would understand that, while the spirit which prompts their devotion and self-sacrifice is praiseworthy, yet the probability of its success is very remote. No doubt there are women who have made this experiment and who have managed to 'reform,' as it is called, confirmed inebriates; but such cases are by no means numerous. While it might not be right to attempt to interfere with any effort to benefit any representative of suffering humanity, it must be remembered that the fate of the next generation is at stake, and that unborn children certainly have rights, although we are very apt to disregard them. Admitting, then, that anyone is at liberty to risk everything, even life itself, to benefit another, nevertheless it cannot be said that anyone has a moral right to jeopardize the future of a family to satisfy any instinct or feeling of affection, however noble it may be. If what I have written is true, no woman is justified in marrying a drunkard."

The unstable nervous organization bequeathed by intemperate parents is like a sword of Damocles over the heads of their unfortunate children, and even moderate drinkers will not give vigorous bodies and strong wills to their descendants. One man boasted that he had used a bottle of wine daily for fifty years, and it had not injured him; but of his twelve children, six died in infancy, one was imbecile, one was insane, the rest were hysterical invalids.

And alcohol is not the only substance that inebriates. Opium, morphine, chloral, cocaine, and all drugs of a similar nature, are dangerous, and each not only inflicts its injury on the individual, but transmits its results to posterity in that nerve degeneration which renders the sufferer an easy victim to all forms of intoxication, and intoxication is nothing more nor less than poisoning. Opium and morphine are often prescribed by physicians, and the patient, experiencing the sudden relief from pain, and perhaps not knowing the danger of indulgence, resorts next time to the delightful pain-quieter on his own responsibility, and almost before he knows it the habit is formed, and the weak will that made the easy victim now makes the unwilling slave, loathing his chains, yet unable to break them; and these evil habits are, in their effects, transmitted.

Dr. Robertson says: "The part that heredity plays in all functional diseases or states of the nervous system is not to be misunderstood. It is safe to assert that no idiopathic case of insanity, chorea, hysteria, megrim, dipsomania, or moral insanity, can occur except by reason of inherited predisposition."

The evils of morphinism are even greater than those of alcoholism, and their transmission no less sure. Especially is there loss of moral power. Dr. Robertson says: "No matter how honorable, upright and conscientious a man's past life may have been, let him become thoroughly addicted to morphine, and I would not believe any statement he might make, either with reference to the use of the drug or on any other subject that concerned his habit. This extends further, and clouds his moral perceptions in all relations of life."

Dr. Brush says: "Cocaine is the only drug the effects of which are more dangerous and more slavish than the inhalation of the fumes of opium."

The danger in the fast life of this age is that we try to find something that will enable us to do our excessive undertakings with less feeling of fatigue. We fail to see in this that we are exhausting our reserve force, instead of adding to our store of force.

The *Popular Science News* says that kola, cocoa, chocolate, coffee, tea, and similar substances make nervous work seem lighter, because they call out the reserve fund which should be most sacredly preserved, and the result is nervous bankruptcy. Understanding that nervous bankruptcy of the parent threatens the welfare of future generations through the law of heredity, we will surely hesitate to bring ourselves under the strain produced by the use of these substances.

The most dangerous habit of the present would almost seem to be the tobacco habit, because it is considered quite respectable and is therefore almost universal. Men who are prominent, not only as statesmen and business men, but also as moral leaders, smoke with no apparent recognition of the evils, and lads can often sanction their beginning of the habit by the fact that a certain pastor or Sunday-school superintendent is a smoker.

But science has not been idle in regard to the investigation of the effects of tobacco, and the discoveries made have been published, so that we are not now ignorant of the tobacco heart, or tobacco throat, or tobacco nerves, nor of the transmission of nerve degeneracy to the children of smokers.

Girls sometimes think it is a great joke to smoke cigarettes for fun, and some grow into the habit of smoking, but the injury is not lessened by the fact that the use of the cigarette was begun in jest, nor that the user is a woman.

In fact, the *Medical Times* is quite inclined to assert that much of the neurasthenia, including a general disturbance of the digestive organs, now so common in that portion of the female sex who have ample means and leisure to indulge in any luxury agreeable to their taste, or which, for the time being, may contribute to their enjoyment, is due to narcotics.

During the Civil War we are told that 13 per cent. of all men examined were excluded as unfit for military service. We are now told that 31 per cent. are found to be unfit. Nearly one-third of the young men found physically incompetent to be soldiers! From what cause? Certainly tobacco must bear a large share of the blame.

Some years ago Major Houston, of the Naval School at Annapolis, made the statement that one-fifth of the boys who applied for admittance were rejected on account of heart disease, and that 90 per cent. of these had produced the heart difficulty by the use of tobacco.

Dr. Pidduch asserts that "the hysteria, the hypochondriasis, the consumption, the dwarfish deformities, the suffering lives and early deaths of the children of inveterate smokers, bear ample testimony to the feebleness of constitution which they have inherited."

Girls sometimes have the idea that a little wildness in a young man is rather to be admired. On one occasion a young woman left a church where she had heard a lecture on the evils of using tobacco, saying, as she went out, "I would not marry a young man if he did not smoke. I think it looks manly, and I don't want a husband who is not a man among men."

Years after, when her three babies died, one after the other, with infantile paralysis, because their father was an inveterate smoker, the habit did not seem to her altogether so admirable, and when she herself became a confirmed invalid, because compelled to breathe night and day a nicotine-poisoned atmosphere, she gave loud voice to her denunciation of the very habit which in her ignorant girlhood she had characterized as manly.

CHAPTER XXIX.

EFFECTS OF IMMORALITY ON THE RACE.

There is another influence at work in causing race degeneracy concerning which the majority of girls are ignorant, and that is immorality. The prevalent idea that young men must "sow their wild oats" is accepted by many young women as true, and they think if the lover reforms before marriage and remains true to them thereafter, that is all they can reasonably demand. They will not make such excuses for themselves for lapses from virtue, but they imbibe the idea that men are not to be held to an absolute standard of purity, and so think it delicate to shut their eyes to the derelictions of young men. This chapter of human life is a sorrowful one to read, but to heed its warnings would save many a girl from sorrow, many a wife from heartache.

The law of God is not a double law, holding woman to the most rigid code of a "thou shalt not" and allowing men the liberty of a "thou mayest."

The penalty inflicted for the violation of moral law is one of the most severe, both in its effects upon the individual transgressor and upon his descendants. The most dreadful scourge of physical disease, as well as moral degeneracy, follows an impure life. This disease, known as syphilis, is practically incurable. It may temporarily disappear, only to reappear in some other form later in life; and even after all signs have become quiescent in the man, they may reappear in his children in some form of transmission. Even one lapse from virtue is enough to taint the young man with this dreadful poison, which may be in after years communicated to his innocent wife or transmitted to his children.

Dr. Guernsey says: "I do not overdraw the picture when I declare that millions of human beings die annually from the effects of poison contracted in this way, in some form of suffering or other; for, by insinuating its effects into and poisoning the whole man, it complicates various disorders and renders them incurable. This horrible infection sometimes becomes engrafted upon other acute diseases, when lingering disorders follow, causing years of misery, and only terminating in death. Sometimes the poison attacks the throat, causing most destructive alterations therein. Sometimes it seizes upon the nasal bones, resulting in their entire destruction and an awful disfigurement of the face. Sometimes it ultimates itself in the ulceration and destruction of other osseous tissues in different portions of the body. Living examples of these facts are too frequently witnessed in the streets of any large city. Young men marrying with the slightest taint of this poison in the blood will surely transmit the disease to their children. Thousands of abortions transpire every year from this cause alone, the poison being so destructive as to kill the child *in utero*, before it is matured for birth; and even if the child be born alive, it is liable to break down with most loathsome disorders of some kind and die during dentition; the few that survive this period are short-lived, and are unhealthy so long as they do live. The first unchaste connection of a man with a woman may be attended with a contamination entailing upon him a life of suffering, and even death itself. Almost imperceptible in its origin, it corrupts the whole body, makes the very air offensive to surrounding friends, and lays multitudes literally to rot in the grave. It commences in one part of the body, and usually, in more or less degree, extends to the whole system, and is said by most eminent physicians to be a morbid poison, having the power of extending itself to every part of the body into which it is infused, and to other persons with whom it in any way comes in contact, so that even its moisture, communicated by linen or otherwise, may corrupt those who unfortunately touch it."

If girls were aware of all this they would not only be careful how they marry immoral men, but they would shrink from personal contact with them as from a viper. Not one, but many girls who have held somewhat lax ideas concerning the propriety of allowing young men to be familiar have reaped the result in a contamination merely through the touch of the lips. To-day a young woman in good social standing is a sufferer from this cause. She was acquainted with a young man of respectable family, but immoral life. His gaiety had a fascination for her, and his reputed wildness only added to the charm. On one evening, as he escorted her home, and took leave of her on the doorstep, she allowed him to kiss her. It chanced that at the time she had a small sore on her lip. The poisonous touch of his lips conveyed the infection through this slight abrasion, and she became tainted with the syphilitic virus, and to-day bears the loathsome disfigurement in consequence. I do not need to multiply such cases. You can be warned by one as well as by a hundred.[2]

A young woman of pure life married a man whose reputation was bad, but whose social position was high. To-day she is suffering from the horrible disease which he communicated to her, and her children have died or are betraying to the world in their very faces the story of their father's wrong deeds. Truly you cannot afford to be ignorant of facts so grave as these.

FOOTNOTES:

[2] For an extended presentation of the character and diseases which accompany vice, the reader is referred to the chapters which treat of this subject in "What a Young Man Ought to Know." Every young woman should be intelligent upon these important subjects. There is nothing in this book to young men which a young woman approaching maturity may not know, both with propriety and benefit, so that she may most successfully protect herself from possible companionship with well-dressed and polite but impure young men by discreetly placing the book in the hands of her father and brothers, that they may become intelligent concerning the dangers against which they can most successfully protect her. It might not be improper for her, after due acquaintance, to see that the book is placed in the hands of the one who seeks to become her husband and the father of her children, that she may at the proper time, and before it is too late, learn whether he has always lived by the standards of social purity which are there set up, and whether he is able to bring to the union the same unsullied life and character which he expects and requires of her.

CHAPTER XXX.

THE GOSPEL OF HEREDITY.

I have often heard people say that God was unjust in making this law of heredity and compelling innocent children to bear the sins of the guilty parents, and at first thought it might so seem; but God is a God of justice and also of mercy, and our study of His laws in their ultimate outcome leads us to know that they are invariably made for our welfare. Let us see, then, if we cannot find something encouraging even in this law of heredity. Are the majority of people born straight or deformed, sick or well, honest or dishonest? You may ask, Are all of these conditions a matter of heredity? Certainly. The fact that we are human beings instead of animals, that we have our due proportion of organs and faculties, that we are not monstrosities or imbeciles, are all hereditary conditions. We see, then, that the law of heredity insures to us our full complement of organs and capabilities, as well as the more pronounced characteristics which we the more readily recognize as inheritances. The fact is that inheritance of good is so universal that we fail to think of it.

When the baby is "well-favored" and straight-limbed, no credit is given to heredity; but if he is in some way out of the ordinary, we blame the law that has fixed on him some result of parental conduct.

If he possesses a good mentality, it scarcely occurs to us that this is just as surely heredity as is the transmission of the mental weakness of some ancestor.

By the Gospel of Heredity I mean this brighter side, this "Good-tidings" of the law. In the first written Biblical record of the law, where the statement is made that the sins of the fathers are visited upon the children to the third and fourth generation, we have also the statement of the "Good-tidings" that the Lord sheweth mercy to thousands of them that love him and keep his commandments; and that means not thousands of individuals, but thousands of generations. Justice is meted to the third and fourth, but mercy to thousands of generations.

All through the Scriptures we find this brighter phase of the law enunciated. Perhaps you would like to study both the law and the Gospel from the Bible. I will give you some texts and you can find them for yourself. It would be interesting also for you to read the lives of men and women of renown, and observe the transmission of talents and capabilities.

Encouraging as this view of the subject may be, it is by no means the brightest side of the subject of heredity, for if we have inherited no special talents, and if we are handicapped by the transmitted results of the sins of our ancestors, we may say "There is no hope for us, nor for our children." To us then will come, as special "Good-tidings of great joy," the news that heredity is not fatality. We are not obliged to sit and quietly bear the fetters our ancestors have forged for us. We can break the chains, we can free ourselves. It may be difficult, but it can be done, and a great incentive to the effort is found in the fact that by success we not only improve ourselves, but we can pass on a better inheritance to our posterity.

We may cultivate our health by obedience to its laws so as to overcome inherited weaknesses to a very great extent. We are not absolutely obliged to die with consumption because one of our parents did. By simple living, and especially by deep breathing of pure air, we may so strengthen ourselves that we will have the power to resist the encroachments of the germ of tuberculosis.

We may be born with weak digestive power, but by plain, wholesome fare, by freedom from worry, by a careful attention to all healthful habits, we may grow strong and free from dyspeptic symptoms.

We can by cultivation of our minds and morals not only increase our own powers, but add to the powers of our posterity.

Then, too, the effects of mental education are transmissible; not the education itself, but an increased capacity, a new tendency. Every mental activity is accompanied by an actual modifying influence on brain structure, so that we are really building our brains by our thoughts, and this increase of our own brains is transmissible to posterity.

I know that some of our philosophers assert strongly that acquired characteristics are not transmitted, and their theories seem quite plausible; but I would rather accept facts than theories any time, and Professor Elmer Gates has demonstrated that this theory does not accord with the facts. He has trained dogs until they could recognize seven or eight shades of green or red. The brains of these dogs, so trained, show under the microscope a great increase of brain-cells in the visual area, proving that the education has created actual brain material. The progeny of these dogs, to several generations, shows at birth a much larger number of brain-cells in the visual area than is the case where the ancestry has not been so strained.

Where the dogs have been brought up in absolute darkness there is a great lack of cells in the visual area, both in these dogs and in their progeny.

This is the brief statement of a most hopeful and encouraging fact.

We look to the dark side of the law of heredity for our warning. It makes us solemnly thoughtful in view of our power over the race in the transmitted result from our own wrongdoing; and then, when we feel overwhelmed and discouraged, we turn towards the Gospel of Heredity and take hope from the fact that good is transmissible; and, more than that, we have it in our power so to modify our own characters, tendencies and habits that we can, in all probability, give our children a better dower than we received, and the earlier in life we begin this making over of ourselves the better.

I have heard people excuse themselves for all manner of faults on the plea that they were inheritances, and therefore could not be overcome. That is to declare that we are slaves, with no chance to acquire freedom, and I am not willing to admit that.

"Whereas in Adam all die, in Christ may all be made alive." That is, that while under the Law of Heredity we are fettered, under the Gospel of Heredity our chains may be broken and we become free.

There is much of encouragement in the poem of Ella Wheeler Wilcox on heredity:

> "There is no trait you cannot overcome.
> Say not thy evil instinct is inherited,
> Or that some trait inborn makes thy whole life forlorn,
> And calls for punishment that is not merited.
>
> "Back of thy parents and grandparents lies
> The great Eternal Will, that, too, is thine
> Inheritance—strong, beautiful, divine;
> Sure lever of success for one who tries.
>
> "Pry up thy fault with this great lever—will;
> However deeply bedded in propensity;
> However firmly set, I tell thee firmer yet
> Is that great power that comes from truth's immensity.
>
> "There is no noble height thou canst not climb;
> All triumphs may be thine in time's futurity,
> If, whatsoe'er thy fault, thou dost not faint or halt,
> But lean upon the staff of God's security.
>
> "Earth has no claim the soul cannot contest;
> Know thyself part of the supernal source,
> And naught can stand before thy spirit's force;
> The soul's divine inheritance is best."

BIBLE TEXTS BEARING ON THE SUBJECT OF HEREDITY.

Natural Heredity.

Law.—Gen. 1:12-24; Ex. 20:6; Num. 14:18.

Sins visited.—Job 21:17-19; Ps. 37:28; Jer. 32:18.

Blessings.—Gen. 22:17, 18; Deut. 4:40; 5:29; 30:19; Ps. 21:13; 37:18, 22, 26, 29; 103:17, 18; 112:1, 2; 128:3; Prov. 10:25; 11:19; 13:22; 17:6; 20:7; Isa. 48:18, 19; Jer. 32:18.

Divine Heredity.

Isa. 43:16; Jer. 3:19; Mal. 2:10; Matt. 5:9, 45, 48; 6:4, 6, 9, 14, 15, 18, 26; John 20:17; Rom. 8:16, 17; Gal. 4:7; Eph. 4:6; 2 Peter 1:4; 1 John 3:2; 5:1.

CHAPTER XXXI.

REQUISITES OF A HUSBAND.

Having spent so much time in the study of principles and laws, we will now return to the discussion of this concrete case. What can you decide in regard to this individual young man to whom you think you have given your heart? What is he in his inheritance? What is he in himself? I do not ask that he shall have inherited wealth, for that often proves a young man's ruin, but does he come of an honest, industrious family? Have you just reason to suppose that he will make a fair success of life? Is his father shiftless, lazy, improvident? If so, it will be harder for him to be provident, business-like. Has he true ideas of the dignity of life and his own responsibility? Is he looking for an "easy job," or does he purpose to give a fair equivalent for all that he receives? Would he rather toil at honest manual labor than be supported by a rich father-in-law?

What are his ideas as to his responsibility in the founding of a home? How will he look upon his wife? As an equal, a companion, or as a plaything, a petted child, or a sort of upper servant? What value does he put upon the wife's labor in the conducting of the household? Will he consider that the money he hands over to her is a gift from him, or only a fair recognition of the value of her work, a rendering to her of her share in the family purse?

What is his estimate of woman? Is she an individual with rights, with intellect and heart, with a judgment to be consulted, opinions worthy of recognition, or only an appendage to man, created for his comfort and to be held in her "sphere" by his will?

What are his defects of temper, or his weaknesses of body? Of course, to you now he seems perfection, and yet he is a human being, fallible and imperfect. If his faults are similar to yours, you double the possibility of their inheritance by your children. If you both have a tendency to lung trouble, the probabilities are that your children will have consumption. If you both are of rheumatic proclivities, you may expect a manifestation of the same early in the life of your children. If you both are "nervous" or irritable in temper, both jealously inclined, or are morbid and melancholy, you need not be surprised at an intensifying of these qualities in your little ones.

If there are more serious family traits, such as insanity, epilepsy, alcoholism and the like, it might even be your duty never to run the risk of their transmission.

I once spoke on heredity when in the audience sat a young man by the side of his *fiancée*, who, I was afterwards told, had been in an insane asylum three times, and yet he purposed marrying her.

I know a clergyman who has wisely dedicated himself to a celibate life because there is marked insanity in his family.

You chafe a little under this reiteration of the duty you owe to children yet unborn, and who may possibly never exist, and perhaps you say, as I have heard girls say, "Oh, I don't mean to have any children;" and perhaps you add, "I don't see why people may not marry and be happy just by themselves without having children."

It is not strange that you should not understand all that is involved in such a statement. It is true that some married people do not have children, and are comparatively happy, and yet perhaps if we could read their hearts we should find that the one great longing of their lives is for the blessing of a child.

It is natural to desire to know the joys of parenthood. In the home, through the cares and love, the anxiety, self-sacrifice, tenderness and patience which accompany parenthood, the education of the individual is made most complete and perfect.

The girl who marries without a willingness to accept these responsibilities is willing to sacrifice that which, rightly borne, will bring her the highest development. If she purposes deliberately to avoid motherhood she puts herself in a position of moral peril, for such immunity is not often secured except at the risk of criminality. I say not often, although I believe that if husband and wife are actuated by the worthy motive of not inflicting on posterity some dower of woe, they are justified in a marriage that does not contemplate parenthood, if they are of lofty purpose enough to live solely in mental and spiritual companionship. But all attempts to secure the pleasure of a physical relation and escape its legitimate results are a menace to the health and a degradation to the moral nature. This subject, and the questions arising therefrom, will be discussed more fully in the next book of this series, "What a Young Wife Ought to Know."

But how is a girl to know all these things concerning her lover's ideas, thoughts, principles, and purposes? Many of these you think cannot be known until after marriage, and then it is too late. That is true; therefore be wise and learn all you can of each other's habits, peculiarities, opinions, and predilections now, before it is too late. Talk over business matters. Find out what your lover's ideas are as to the wife's right to a pecuniary recognition of the value of her labor in making the home. Does he think that she earns nothing, and that what he gives her of his money is a donation for which she gives no return? I know a young woman who had been self-supporting before her marriage who felt timid about asking her husband for money. So she wore her wedding garments until they were shabby, went without money when her own funds were exhausted, and kept silent for five years, and her husband—a young clergyman—never thought to ask her if she needed anything, never observed her growing shabbiness. When at last she summoned courage to tell him her needs, he was overwhelmed with regret for his own lack of thought and observation, and yet he could not understand why she should hesitate to ask for money. "Why, it is all yours, dear," he said. "You were only asking for what already belongs to you." And many young husbands are just as obtuse, therefore they should receive in advance the instruction that is needed to prevent a possibility of such neglect. Have it understood that if you are worthy to be trusted as a bearer of the name and a sharer of the fortunes of a man, you are worthy to share also the burden of the knowledge of his business experiences, and to bear the responsibility of economically guarding his interests in the expenditure of money which, by your love and care and labor, you have helped him to earn.

I think a young woman should know something of the personal habits of her future husband. Does he like fresh air, or does he want the windows hermetically sealed at night. Is he a believer in the godliness of cleanliness? I have just read of two people who married after a six week's acquaintance, knowing nothing of each other's antecedents, personal habits, caprices or principles. The man proved to be a regular hypochondriac, taking medicine constantly, at one time with five doctors prescribing for him. He counted his pulse at every odd moment, and looked at his tongue instead of at the eyes of his wife, as he had done when a lover. He had a dread of pure air, and was as averse to bathing as a cat. The woman had lived in the open air, taken a daily morning bath, and was disgusted with those who did not do likewise. The writer says, "She stormed, took her baths, and opened the windows; he cried, took no baths, shut the windows, and called the doctors." There is no need to depict the unhappiness of the home, and yet no doubt the girl would have been shocked had anyone suggested that she inquire into these facts concerning her lover. But if she had been less romantic and more practical, if she had remembered that the marriage contract would bind her for life to one who would be more closely connected with her than anyone else could be, and this union for life, by day and by night, constant, continuous, and not to be annulled by any such small matters as bad breath or unpleasant personal habits, perhaps she would have considered it no small matter to discover the possible causes of disgust before they became fixtures in her life.

And perhaps, also, she would have given her own personal habits more consideration. True love will endure much, but it sometimes dies in the presence of untidiness, of carelessness as to dress or room, or lack of sweetness of person or of breath. If you demand much of a husband, he has a right to demand just as much from you. If there are habits concerning which you would rather he as a lover should be ignorant, believe me that it is even more important that as a husband he should not know them. Therefore employ your available time before marriage to rid yourself of them. If a lover would be disenchanted to see the room from which his blooming, beauteous adored one had departed, bearing the marks of carelessness and disorder, with soiled clothing, unmade bed, shoes, hose and dresses all in tumbled heaps on chairs and floor, remember that the marriage ceremony does not make such a room more attractive to the husband, who must not only see but share its discomforts.

In addition to the knowledge of each other's personal peculiarities there should be an understanding of each other's ideas as to the duties and responsibilities of their proposed relation to each other. I lately received a letter from a young woman who asks, "How freely do you think two engaged young people may talk concerning their future life? Would it not be indelicate for them to discuss their future relations, the possibility and responsibilities of parenthood, etc.?"

I answer, that depends on the young people. If they have false ideas, if they have little or no scientific knowledge, if their thoughts are filled with wrong mental pictures, they will not know how to talk wisely and beneficially. But these two young people are intelligent, are scientifically educated, are Christians. Their hearts are pure, their standards high, their motives praiseworthy. It would seem that they might talk as freely as their inclination would prompt. In fact there seems to me more indelicacy and more danger from long evenings spent in murmuring ardent protestations of love and indulging in embraces and endearments than in a frank, serious conversation on the realities and responsibilities of marriage, an exchange of earnest thoughts, voiced in chaste, well-chosen language—a conversation which by its very solemnity is lifted out of the realm of sense-pleasure into the dignified domain of science and morality.

CHAPTER XXXII.

ENGAGEMENTS.

There now sparkles on your finger a ring that symbolizes the promise you have given to become a wife. You are engaged, and there now arises in your mind the query as to the conduct of yourselves during this period of engagement: How much of privilege shall you grant your lover? As you are promised to each other for life, are you not warranted in assuming towards each other greater personal familiarity? May you not with perfect modesty allow endearments and caresses that hitherto have not been permissible?

I take it for granted that you are not one of those unwise young women who permit themselves to become engaged for fun; who consider an engagement as of so little seriousness that it may be made and broken without regret. I have known girls who even enter into engagements just in order to feel justified in greater freedom of conduct without compunction of conscience. If such engagements do not violate the code of conventionalities they certainly infringe upon the moral code.

It is not strange that girls should fail to see all the dangers of such conduct—that they should not comprehend that thus they become sources of temptation to their lovers, and may even imperil their own safety.

But your engagement is an honest one, your love is true, based upon thorough acquaintance; you have mutual respect and entire confidence in each other. May you not now throw aside much of the restrictions that have surrounded your association and manifest your affection in reciprocal demonstrations?

We often read the advice to young people not to enter upon long engagements, and the reason given is that it exacts too much in the way of self-control, is too great a nervous strain, is too full of peril. I would like to quote just here a few words by Dr. C.W. Eaton:

"Away with the sexual argument against engagements, and let us all set about that cultivation of will and purpose which can make the weakest a tower of strength and the arbiter of his own destiny; and let us say to our appetites, Thus far shalt thou come and no farther, neither shalt thou presume to deny to thy master the best earthly companionship which may come into his life. It may be a far harder task than the ardent and poetical lover allows himself at first to think, but the hardest battles are best worth the fighting; and what manner of men should we become if we systematically evaded life's conflicts, instead of meeting them squarely and fighting them through manfully? Dr. Bourgeois says: 'The ancient custom of betrothals is the safeguard for the purity of morals and the happy association of man and wife. This institution was known to the Greeks, the Hebrews, the Romans, and during the Middle Ages. In Germany it has still preserved its poetical and moral character. The young people are sometimes affianced many years before their marriage. We see the young man, thus betrothed, with heart full of his chaste love, absent himself for a time in order to finish his education, to perform his studies of science or art, his apprenticeship to a trade, and to prepare himself for manly life. He returns to his betrothed with a soul which has remained pure, with a reason enlarged and fortified. Then both are ripe for the austere duties of marriage.

"'Chaste love, consecrated by betrothals, can be cultivated in the midst of work. It lightens toil, it banishes *ennui*, it illumines the horizon of life with delightful prospects; it excites in the young man the manly courage and the high intelligence to create for himself a position in the world; in woman, the noble ambition to perfect herself to become a worthy companion and good adviser.

"'During the stormy period of youth it is the only means of preserving the virgin purity of the heart and of the body. Does anyone believe that young men who in good season have in their hearts a love strong and worthy of them would profane themselves, as they so often otherwise do, in vile affections, in those relations of a day, giving themselves a holocaust to beauty without soul, or even to licentiousness without beauty?'"

What a Young Woman Ought to Know

Emerson says: "If, however, from too much conversing with material objects the soul was gross, and misplaced its satisfaction in the body, it reaped nothing but sorrow, body being unable to fulfill the promise which beauty holds out; but if, accepting the hint of these visions and suggestions which beauty makes to his mind, the soul passes through the body and fails to admire strokes of character, and the lovers contemplate one another in their discourses and their actions, then they pass to the true palace of beauty, more and more inflame their love of it, and by this love extinguishing the base affection, as the sun puts out fire by shining on the hearth, they become pure and hallowed. By conversation with that which is in itself excellent, magnanimous, lowly and just, the lover comes to a warmer love of these nobilities, and a quicker apprehension of them. Then he passes from loving them in one to loving them in all, and so is the one beautiful soul only the door through which he enters to the society of all true and pure souls. In the particular society of his mate he attains a clearer sight of any spot, any taint which her beauty has contracted from this world, and is able to point it out, and this with mutual joy that they are now able, without offense, to indicate blemishes and hindrances in each other, and give to each all help and comfort in curing the same. And beholding in many souls the traits of the divine beauty, and separating in each soul that which is divine from the taint which it has contracted in the world, the lover ascends to the highest beauty, to the love and knowledge of the Divinity, by steps on this ladder of created souls."

And this all means that when the thought of the sex-relation constitutes in the mind of either the idea of marriage, then the wedding ceremony will be supposed to remove all restrictions, and the only limit of gratification will be the limit of desire. Under these circumstances the close familiarity of a long engagement would be a mental and physical tax, because the self-control exercised is felt to be only temporary, and will be no longer needed when the wedding ceremony has been said.

But if the idea of marriage is nobler, if the sex-relation is consecrated to its highest purpose of reproduction, if marriage is felt to be only an added opportunity for self-control, which will be more difficult then because there will be no restraint except that which is self-imposed, then the engagement will be felt to be a time of gradual preparation for that closer relationship which needs more will-power because opportunity is greater.

Under these conditions the lovers will be aiming towards an ideal which recognizes that in wedded life all that is lasting in affection, in tender courtesy, in most intimate companionship, in sweetest demonstration, is possible without the physical union, which in itself is the most transitory of pleasures, but which in unlimited indulgence becomes the most domineering of passions, exhaustive of physical power and of mental vigor, and absolutely annihilating all true love.

If you ask why there should exist this marvelous drawing of the sexes towards each other if their relation is not based upon the exercise of sex-functions, I reply that sex is more than its local expression; it is inherent in mind as well as body, and therefore sexual power may be expressed in masculine courage, energy or daring, or in feminine constancy, self-abnegation, or sweet courtesy. Sexual attraction is not limited to the local expression, nor creative power to reproduction of kind, but may give a stimulus to the intellectual companionship of men and women, and result in the creation of nobler ideals and grander aspirations.

Having settled in your mind your attitude towards your lover, let us consider what it shall be towards your family during these days of the engagement. Naturally you will not feel a separation from the home circle as keenly as do the other members of your family. You two are so absorbed in each other, are so busy exchanging ideas, in becoming acquainted, that you are oblivious to the change brought about in your family. You think you two ought to be allowed the privilege of *tête-à-têtes*, for of course you cannot talk freely together in the hearing of others. This is true. You should have times of seclusion, when, without a sense of oppression through fear of criticism or jesting, you can rhapsodize, or quote poetry and open your hearts' treasures to each other. But you still owe a duty to your home. Doubtless your mother is not now as necessary to your happiness as you are to hers. She is thinking of you with most tender solicitude, she misses your presence, she already begins to feel the loneliness of the inevitable separation. If you are thoughtful you will see to it that the separation does not begin sooner than is necessary. Then, too, your parents need to get acquainted with this new member whom you are to introduce into the family, and he needs to know them. He will think none the less of you if he sees that you do not allow him to monopolize you entirely, that you recognize your obligations to the family and that you expect him to recognize them also, and, in addition, his obligations to show them due courtesy and attention. He is not to absorb you entirely, to take you out of the home circle, but he is to come in and be a part of it, even as you are to become one in the home of which he is a member. You need to remember that he is son and brother to women who loved him long before you knew him, and that he still owes them attention and thoughtful, affectionate courtesy.

Never allow yourself to feel jealous of his mother or sisters. The fact that he is a loving, thoughtful son and brother is in a measure a guarantee that he will be a loving, thoughtful husband.

Let me add to this advice a word more. Do not allow yourself to feel jealous of him in any way. Jealousy is the quintessence of selfishness, and no other passion is so destructive of happiness, so full of the contagion of evil. If your lover is not to be trusted, you would be wise to end the engagement at once. If he is to be trusted, that trust should be absolute. I said you should not allow him to monopolize you, neither should you attempt to monopolize him. There are other people in the world besides yourself, and other occupations than the business of waiting on you. If you make him feel that he dare not speak to anyone but you, that he dare not think of anything but you, he will begin to chafe under the restraint and feel a desire to break the bonds that are becoming fetters. If he were not your acknowledged lover, if you were anxious to win his love, but were a little uncertain as to your power to do so, you would not meet him with tears and upbraidings because he had for one moment seemed to forget you, but you would at once use every possible effort to make yourself more attractive in his eyes than any other person could possibly be. You will be wise to use those same tactics now, even though his allegiance is pledged to you. Be so charming that no one else can be considered so entertaining; that no one else can be so wise, so witty, so sympathetic, so altogether lovely, that everything but yourself is forgotten; and then believe in him so absolutely that he could not possibly swerve in his fidelity to you. Have you ever thought that to accuse one of a certain wrong act may be just the way to suggest to him the possibility of committing it? If one trusts you implicitly, that very trust is a constant suggestion to be true, and doubt is a suggestion to act worthy of being doubted.

You must trust each other or you have no sure foundation for future love and happiness. It needs a great deal of good common sense to learn how to live happily in marriage. You may have chosen wisely. The man may be honest, pure, kindly, intelligent, and Christian, but he is human, therefore not perfect. He has faults, peculiarities, moods, perhaps tempers, and he will probably not wait until you are married to begin to show them. There will come differences of opinions, divergences in desires, clashings in judgment. Now is the time to display your tact, to learn how to express an opposing opinion without arousing antagonism, to yield a desire for the sake of a greater love than that of self, to adhere to principle without unpleasant discussion; in short, to be dignified and womanly without pettiness or littleness of any kind. You remember the words of Ruskin, that the woman must be "incorruptibly good, instinctively, infallibly wise, not for self-development, but for self-renunciation," and that will be the highest development.

No doubt you will think that some of this advice should be given to young men as well as to young women, and I think so too, and were I talking to your lover I could say many warning words; but just now I am telling you things that he does not need to hear, and I do not need to tell you what, if I had the chance, I would say to him. You are to train yourself and not him, and yet I would not have you ignorant of your power over him in developing in him all that is noblest and best. You should hold him ever to his highest ideals. He should never feel so absolutely sure of your adoration as to imagine that it will endure a lowering of his standards. You have been posing a little before each other. Doubtless you were not aware of this, but, now that you have each gained the heart of the other, you may sometimes feel that you can relax; but this is a dangerous error. You should continue to be as thoughtful, as courteous, as careful as ever;

you should endeavor really to be all that you have tried or appeared to be during these days of courtship. You will be none too perfect even then.

Once, in talking to a group of women, I asserted that a wife should exact of her husband as high a tone of morality as of her lover, that she should not allow him to become lax in his conversation with her any more than with any other woman. One woman thought me too strict. She said men liked to feel that at home they could do as they pleased, and would resent a wife's interference with their right to be loose in their talk in their own home. I replied that the home is not the man's nor the woman's alone; it is theirs jointly; that each has a right to demand that the other shall not pollute or poison the air, the food, the water or the moral atmosphere; and the wife who allows contamination of the thought-atmosphere of the home is as culpable as if she were to permit poison to be put into the food.

As a man admires the girl who respects herself too much to permit him to tell her questionable stories, so will he reverence the wife who refuses to allow him to degrade himself in her presence either by speech or conduct. Love would not so often fail if wives knew the secret of retaining it, and that is not by sacrifice of principle, nor by tearful reproaches and upbraidings, but by being true to the highest impulses, and while having the good common sense that can make all reasonable allowance for fallibility, still permits no lowering of moral standards, no willful falling short of the very best.

CHAPTER XXXIII.

THE WEDDING.

Said my friend:

There's to be a grand wedding, you know,
With no end to the fuss and parade,
With sixteen fair bridesmaids to stand in a row,
With sixteen young groomsmen to help out the show,
One to stand by the side of each maid.

Then there's a reception to be very fine,
With all sorts of magnificent things,
With silver to glitter and mirrors to shine,
With tropical fruit and famous old wine,
With odorous flowers and music divine,
Drawn forth from melodious strings.

In the minds of many girls the wedding means only this public show, the display of elegant toilets, the reception of costly gifts; and the preparation of marriage means too often merely the making of an elegant *trousseau*. People generally do not ask concerning the fitness of the young people to enter on the solemn duties of life—do not ask how well they have been instructed concerning that which is before them; but the questions are all about clothes and gifts and ceremonials. No wonder, then, that the thought of the young woman centers on these things, to the exclusion of nearly all else; indeed, it may be to the detriment of health and the lessening of true happiness. The prospective husband finds his *fiancée* so absorbed in sewing, shopping and interviews with dressmakers that she has few moments to give to him, and these few occupied more with the thought of gowns and personal adornments than with ideals of wedded happiness.

Perhaps she even excuses herself for lessening the number of his visits on the plea that very soon now she will be all his, and so he is left to spend his last days of bachelorhood in loneliness, and made to feel that raiment is more than love. Worse still, it may be that on the wedding-day he takes to his heart a bride so wearied, so nervously exhausted by the preparations of the *trousseau* that she is at least temporarily an invalid. I have known more than one bride so worn out by the preparation for her wedding that instead of bringing brightness, joy and beauty into the new life, she brought illness, anxiety and care, and made demands at once upon the patience and service of the husband, who had a right to expect health and vigor and a power to enjoy.

I knew a sensible girl who said months before her marriage, "I am not going to bring to my new life a remnant of health, a shattered nervous system and a tattered temper," and she kept her word. Her sewing was done by degrees, and was all out of the way weeks before the wedding. Shopping and dressmaking were never allowed to interfere with the walks and drives, the chats and moonlight strolls. "We shall not be able to repeat this experience," she wisely said, and so her lover found her ever ready to give him her society and her thought. Her *trousseau* was not elaborate, her wedding-dress was simple, but in it she shone like a flower of the morning, full of brightness and health and joy.

She was wise in other respects. Only her intimate friends were invited to the wedding ceremony, and to these she said, "I want you to feel that it is you I invite, not your gifts. If your love impels you to give me some simple memento of yourself it will be cherished, but I'd rather have a pincushion made by your own hand, or a little flower painted by yourself, than the most costly purchased picture or most elegant piece of silver that you bought, because you thought it was expected. And if, when you come, you bring no gift but your love and blessing, I shall feel that that is the richest treasure."

There was no display of presents to a vulgar curiosity, no collection of duplicate butter-knives or berry-spoons to be secretly disposed of after the wedding. The gifts were few and not costly, but each told its own story of personal affection, and therefore really had a meaning.

This sensible young woman introduced another innovation into her wedding. She would not listen to the suggestion of a bridal tour. "I do not want to be stared at and commented on by strangers," she said. "Let us go to some quiet spot in the mountains or by the sea, and let us live with each other and with nature." In after years she often said, "I would not miss from my memory the picture of those happy days for anything that any trip on railway trains and sojourns at hotels could give me. We had time and opportunity to learn each other's souls as we could not have done amid 'the madding crowd;' and we have loved each other more truly, I know, because in those early wedded days we sat with Nature and Nature's God in the true companionship which such solitude alone can bring."

I never see the parade of a fashionable wedding that I am not reminded of her and of a sad contrast to her experience, when two young people were married amid a blaze of light, a rain of flowers, and under the curious eyes of hundreds of strangers took their wedding tour, while the papers glowingly described the dress and beauty of the bride, the necktie and the trousers of the groom, and pictures of the two were labeled "The Happy Couple." In two years the bride came home to her parents wrecked in health and broken in heart.

There is a beauty in a golden wedding that truly celebrates a happy union of half a century. But when life is all untried, when perhaps the two young people know nothing of what is before them, it may be are but little acquainted with each other, and have mistaken the thrill of passion for the steady exaltation of love, then it would seem wiser to make the occasion one of most solemn import, free from glitter and show, and full of that deep meaning which makes the heart stand still in reverence for life's deepest mysteries.

> O, gallant young groom, it may seem a slight thing
> To take this young girl as your bride;
> To place on her finger the plain golden ring,
> Around her these bright flower-festoons to fling,
> But have you e'er thought what the future will bring
> To you in this life so untried?
>
> Have you thought how your temper may often be tried?
> That you may grow gouty and old,
> That the fair smiling face of your bonnie young bride

What a Young Woman Ought to Know

May grow pale and haggard, and wrinkled, beside,
Or she prove a sloven and scold?

And you, bonnie bride, on this glad wedding day,
In the midst of the curious crowd,
Do you fancy that life will be always so gay?
Can you work, can you wait, do you know how to pray,
Can you suffer, and not cry aloud?

Can you watch out the hours by sad beds of pain?
Can you bear and forbear and forgive?
Can you cheerfully hope e'en when hoping is vain,
And when hope is dead, and to die you would fain,
Can you still feel it right you should live?

O, touchingly solemn and tender the hour,
So full of deep meaning the vow
You have uttered. And sorely you need Divine power
To guide you and guard you in sunshine and shower,
For trouble will come and love's delicate flower
Be crushed, you can scarcely tell how.

And yet, dear heart, there is nothing that has such unconquerable vitality as love; but it must be true love, not self-love, not sentimentality, not passion, not any of the spurious emotions that masquerade under the name of love, and which wither with the slightest adverse wind.

Love is not an exotic, growing only in the conservatories of wealth. It is a hardy plant, covering desolate places with verdure, glowing amid the snows of mountain peaks, blossoming by night as well as by day, hiding defects, clinging to ruins, enduring drouth and heat and cold.

I know a woman who says that there should never be marriage where there are unpleasant peculiarities, idiosyncrasies, or even mannerisms; but should we act on that principle, few would marry. Love is sometimes said to be blind in the days of wooing, but wearing magnifying glasses after wedlock. True love is never blind, but he is capable of judging of true relative values, and will count as naught the slight defect when measured by the overwhelming perfection. Who has not seen men devoted to wives who were homely or peculiar, but who were genuinely pure and true?

"I don't care," said one woman, "if my husband is bald and cross-eyed, he has a heart of gold."

True love is not blind, but with a deep, keen insight looks through the encasing garment of human imperfections, and sees within the divine ego, and because it recognizes the true inner self that is worthy, hopeth all things, believeth all things, endureth all things, and never faileth.

THE END.

What a Young Woman Ought to Know

Offices *of* Publication

¶ IN THE UNITED STATES. The Vir Publishing Company, 200-214 N. Fifteenth St., Philadelphia, Pa.

¶ IN ENGLAND. The Vir Publishing Company, 4 Imperial B'l'd'g's, Ludgate Circus, London, E.C.

¶ IN CANADA. Ryerson Press, Cor. Queen and John Sts. Toronto, Ontario.

"What a Young Girl Ought to Know."

BY MRS. MARY WOOD-ALLEN, M.D.

Condensed Table of Contents

PART I

The origin of life—One plan in all forms of life—How plants grow from the seed—They feed on the soil, grow and mature—How the plant reproduces itself—The flower, the pollen, the pod, the seed—The office of bees and insects in fertilization.

PART II

Fishes and their young—The parent fishes and the baby fishes—The seeds of plants and eggs of fishes, birds and animals—How fishes never know their baby offspring—Warm blooded animals—Lessons from birds—Their nests, eggs and little ones.

PART III

Animals and their young—The place which God has prepared for their young—Beginning their independent life—Human babies the

What a Young Woman Ought to Know

most helpless and dependent of all creatures—The relations of parent and child—The child a part of each parent—Heredity and its lessons.

PART IV

The value of good health—The care of the body—The body a temple to be kept holy—Girls should receive their instruction from their mothers—The body the garment which the soul wears—Effects of thoughts upon life and character—Value of good companions, good books and good influences—What it is to become a woman.

"What a Young Girl Ought to Know"

WHAT EMINENT PEOPLE SAY

Francis E. Willard, LL.D.

"I do earnestly hope that this book, founded on a strictly scientific but not forgetting a strong ethical basis, may be well known and widely read by the dear girls in their teens and the young women in their homes."

Mrs. Elizabeth B. Grannis

"These facts ought to be judiciously brought to the intelligence of every child whenever it asks questions concerning its own origin."

Mrs. Harriet Lincoln Coolidge

"It is a book that mothers and daughters ought to own."

Mrs. Katharine L. Stevenson

"The book is strong, direct, pure, as healthy as a breeze from the mountain-top."

What a Young Woman Ought to Know

Mrs. Isabelle MacDonald Alden, "Pansy"

"It is just the book needed to teach what most people do not know how to teach, being scientific, simple and plain-spoken, yet delicate."

Miss Grace H. Dodge

"I know of no one who writes or speaks on these great subjects with more womanly touch than Mrs. Wood-Allen, nor with deeper reverence. When I listen to her I feel that she has been inspired by a Higher Power."

Ira D. Sankey

"Every mother in the land that has a daughter should secure for her a copy of "What a Young Girl Ought to Know." It will save the world untold sorrow."

"What a Young Wife Ought to Know."

BY MRS. EMMA F.A. DRAKE, M.D.

Condensed Table of Contents

HUSBAND AND HOME

The choice of a husband—One worthy of both love and respect—Real characteristics necessary—Purity vs. "wild oats"—What shall a young wife expect to be to her husband?—His equal, but not his counterpart—His helpmeet Wifehood and motherhood—Should keep pace with his mental growth—Trousseau and wedding presents—The foolish and ruinous display at weddings—Wedding presents and unhappiness—Wise choice of furniture—The best adornments for the home.

THE MARITAL RELATIONS

The marital state should be the most holy of sanctuaries—Its influence upon character—Modesty—Reproduction the primal purpose—Love's highest plane—The right and wrong of marriage—The wrongdoings of good men.

PARENTHOOD

Preparation for motherhood—Motherhood the glory of womanhood—Maternity productive of health—Clothing—Exercise—Baths, etc., etc.—The child the expression of the mother's thoughts—The five stages of prenatal culture.

PREPARATION FOR FATHERHOOD

Questions which test the fitness of young men for marriage—Many young men of startling worth—Effects of bad morals and wayward habits—Tobacco and Alcoholics—Attaining the best—The father reproduced in his children.

ANTENATAL INFANTICIDE

The moral responsibility of parents in heredity—The mother's investment of moulding power—Parents workers together with God—Ailments during expectant motherhood—Maternity a normal state—Development of the fœtus—Minuteness of the germ of human life—Changes which take place—Life present the moment conception takes place—The sin of tampering with the work of the Infinite.

THE LITTLE ONE

Baby's wardrobe—The question that comes with fluttering signs of life—Importance of wise choice of material and style of dress—Choice of physician and nurse of real consequence—The birth chamber—Surroundings and after-care of the mother—The care of the baby—The responsibilities and joys of motherhood—The mother the baby's teacher—Common ailments of children and how to treat them—Guarding against vice—The training of children—Body building—Helps for mothers.

"What a Young Wife Ought to Know"

WHAT EMINENT PEOPLE SAY

Mrs. Margaret E. Sangster

"Joyfully I send you my unqualified endorsement of the excellent book, 'What a Young Wife Ought to Know.' I wish every young and perplexed wife might read its pages."

Charles H. Parkhurst, D.D.

"It handles delicate matters in a manner as firm as it is delicate, and dignifies even what is common by the purity of the sentiment and nobility of intent with which it is treated."

Marietta Holly (Josiah Allen's Wife)

"It is an excellent book; if every young wife of to-day would read it and lay its lessons to heart it would make the to-morrow much easier and happier for all of Eve's daughters."

W.G. Sperry, M.D.

"Young wives, for whom this book is intended, wilt receive great benefits from heeding its wise words. It is good for incitement, guidance, restraint."

Mrs. Joseph Cook

"It illuminates the Holy of Holies in the most sacred of earthly relationships with the white light of truth and purity."

What a Young Woman Ought to Know

Julia Holmes Smith, M.D.

"Be sure Dr. Drake's book is part of your daughter's outfit. I have never read anything which so thoroughly met the use it was designed for as this volume."

J.P. Sutherland, M.D.

"A subject difficult to treat has been handled by Dr. Drake with delicacy, earnestness and straightforwardness. It is a practical book destined to do good."

"What a Woman of Forty-five Ought to Know."

BY MRS. EMMA F.A. DRAKE, M.D.

Condensed Table of Contents

KNOWLEDGE OF CLIMACTERIC NECESSARY

Why women are not prepared to meet the climacteric—The fear that unnerves many—Error of views concerning "Change of Life"—Correct teaching stated—Influence of medical literature—Three periods in a woman's life—Relation of early habits to later aches and ills—The menopause—Conditions which influence the period of the climacteric—The age at-which it usually appears—Effects of heredity—Childless women—Mothers of large families—Effects of different occupations—Excesses.

HERALDS OF CHANGE—DISEASES AND REMEDIES

Mental states during menopause—Change in blood currents—Flushes, chilliness, dizziness, etc.—Nervous symptoms—Disturbed mental and nervous equilibriums—Nature as woman's helper—Troublesome ailments—Mental troubles considered—Suggested help—Cancer—Benefits named—Apprehensions dispelled—How to banish worry—Simplifying daily duty—An eminent physician's

What a Young Woman Ought to Know

prescription—A word to single women—Reluctance of unmarried women to meet the menopause—How to prolong one's youth—Dress during this period—The mother "At Sea"—Guarding against becoming gloomy—Effects of patent medicine advertising—Drug fiends—Lustful indulgence.

WHAT BOTH HUSBAND AND WIFE SHOULD REMEMBER

Slights and inattentions keenly felt by her—Need of patience—A word of private counsel—Value of little attentions—Wife's duty to her husband—Holding husband's affections—Making home attractive—Unselfishness.

AUTO-SUGGESTION AND OTHER SUGGESTIONS

Influence of mind over body—The mind as a curative agent—How to rise out of depression—Mental philosophy and physical betterment—Relation of health to sight—Care of the teeth—The hair—Constipation—Self cure—Choice of foods—Exercise—Physical development—Exercise of mind and soul.

"What a Woman of Forty-five Ought to Know"

PRAISED BY THE PRESS

"Will dispel apprehensions aroused by groundless forebodings."—*Reformed Church Messenger.*

"If the hygienic advice in this book is followed it will lengthen the lives of women and make their closing years the happiest and most useful of all,"—*Herald and Presbyter.*

"In no line of literature, perhaps, is such a book so much needed."—*New Haven Leader.*

"Those who peruse the book only from prurient curiosity will be disappointed."—*Cleveland World.*

"Should be read by every woman nearing and passing middle life." —*Pittsburg Gazette.*

"Written in that wholesome sympathetic manner characteristic of all the books in the Self and Sex Series." —*Cleveland Daily World.*

"Full of most admirable practical advice, and it is written in a sympathetic manner which is the outcome of oneness of sex between the author and those whom she addresses." —*Syracuse Herald.*

"There are some things that a woman of forty-five does not know — things which she regards with more or less terror in the expectation — which terror it is the object of Mrs. Drake to dispel." —*Rochester Herald.*

"There is nothing in the book that could not be proclaimed from the house-tops, and there is everything in it that intelligent and thoughtful women should read and keep for their daughters to read when the proper time comes." —*Newark Daily Advertiser.*

A New Book by Charles Frederic Goss

More Important than the Simple or the Strenuous Life is the Home Life

"HUSBAND, WIFE AND HOME"

By CHARLES FREDERIC GOSS

Author of "The Redemption of David Corson," etc., etc.

"This is the kind of book that one desires to read aloud to all the family. Its captivating stories, humorous often, pathetic at times, will brighten one's face into a broad smile or bring the tear unbidden. The stories are the windows that Dr. Goss opens upon the practical themes that brighten every page of this winsome book. It will drive away the "blues" and make a cross and glum person look pleasant and feel pleasant. The divorce courts would be forced to go out of business if its blessed home truths were put into practice."

ENTHUSIASTICALLY ENDORSED BY THE PRESS

"There are nearly fifty short chapters. It boxes the compass of its subject, skipping no point. Wide experience and keen observation of real life yield material which is treated with plain, common sense, good wit and no lack of humor. Thus it hits the need of the average man and woman, and all others that reckon themselves above the average. The whole book is pervaded by strong and pure moral feeling, and the chapters are well dotted with pithy anecdotes and amusing stories." —*The Outlook.*

"These talks are practical, pungent and full of the sap of experience." —*Bookseller, Newsdealer and Stationer.*

"The call of the hour is for such a book as this to be read and heeded. Every chapter is on a subject bound to come up sooner or later, and discussed plainly but from a high Christian standpoint." —*Religious Telescope.*

"This book is a wholesome, exceedingly digestible oatmeal of literature which is better for the mental and moral stomach than many a higher-flavored repast." —*St. Louis Republic.*

Price, $1.50 net, post free

A NEW DEVOTIONAL BOOK

"Faces Toward the Light"

By Sylvanus Stall, D.D.

Every phase of the Christian life—its joys and sorrows, its temptations and triumphs—is treated in a reverent and deeply spiritual manner that is sure to prove helpful and inspiring to every reader.

SOME CHAPTERS IN THE BOOK

Glory After Gloom. The Dangerous Hour. The Concealed Future. Gleaning for Christ. Hunger and Health. Direction and Destiny. God of the Valleys. Coins and Christians. Reserved Blessings. Comfort in Sorrow. The Better Service. Not Knowing Whither. Good, but Good for Nothing. No Easy Place. The Dead Prayer Office. How God Reveals Himself. Starting Late. Source of Power. Toiling at a Heavy Tow. What He Gave and What He Got. Vacation Lessons. Wheat or Weeds. The Christian's Power. Disclosures in the Cloud. Healing and Living Waters. The Concealed Future. Suspended Animation. The Source of Power. Lessons from the Leaves. Etc.

Just Published.   New Revised Edition.

FIVE-MINUTE OBJECT SERMONS TO CHILDREN

Through Eye-Gate and Ear-Gate Into the City of Child-Soul

By SYLVANUS STALL, D.D.

A book for preachers, teachers, parents and all interested in the training and culture of children.

ENTHUSIASTICALLY COMMENDED

"These little delightful sermons are models at point and brevity, and reach the little hearts through the eye and ear." —*Christian Observer.*

"Boys and girls will devour every one of them with relish, whilst we children of a larger growth will be children again." —*Lutheran Observer.*

"These sermons cannot help being suggestive to every preacher who would interest children, and they also have a much wider scope than for the pulpit. The book should be eagerly sought by all Sunday-School Teachers, leaders of children's meetings and the clergymen of all churches." —*Wesleyan Methodist.*

"Dr. Stall has the happy faculty of presenting to children, sober truths in a manner interesting to them. The author's object is to implant in the child's mind seeds of truth and love, nobleness and justice, and all the virtues that go to make a manly boy and womanly girl, as well as a God-loving child." —*Boston Times.*

Talks to the King's Children

Second Series of "Five-Minute Object Sermons"
By SYLVANUS STALL, D.D.

Invaluable in THE HOME, THE SUNDAY SCHOOL, THE PASTOR'S LIBRARY, THE MISSION FIELD

A CHILDREN'S PREACHER

"Dr. Stall has few equals in this particular line of writing. He shows a fine reserve in not allowing the object used to overshadow the truth taught." —*Nashville Christian Advocate.*

"The Rev. Dr. Sylvanus Stall is one of the best preachers for young people in the American pulpit. His 'Five-minute Object Sermons' to children was an ideal book in its class. The present volume is a second series of the same kind, and will be found to have no less point and charm than the volume published two years ago." —*New York Independent.*

"The author is well-known in this community, having been a pastor in Baltimore City for several years. He is an adept certainly in furnishing bright, interesting talks to children. He writes with a vigorous, irresistible pen." —*Baltimore Methodist.*

THE CHILDREN GOOD JUDGES

"Those who have had the genuine pleasure and profit of Dr. Stall's first series of children's sermons will welcome this second volume. We have read them with the children and commend them very highly. The children know a good sermon when they hear it."—*Reformed Church Messenger.*

"Irresistibly interesting, especially to the young mind."—*Christian Work.*

JUST PUBLISHED

Two Important Booklets

By Mrs. Adolphe Hoffmann, who is widely known in France, Germany and Switzerland as a talented writer, lecturer and educator. She is also prominent in the great reform and educational movements in Europe.

The Social Duty of Our Daughters

A mother's talk with mothers and their grown daughters.

BY MRS. ADOLPHE HOFFMANN

An affectionate and confidential talk to mothers and their daughters on the responsibility, power and maternal duties of woman. These counsels should do much to dignify and elevate parenthood to the place intended by the Creator.

What a Young Woman Ought to Know

Before Marriage

A mother's parting counsel to her son on the eve of his marriage.

BY MRS. ADOLPHE HOFFMANN

This booklet embodies the counsel of an earnest mother who imparts to her son the information essential to the happiness both of her son and his bride.

Unique   Original   Uplifting

God's Minute

A book of 365 daily prayers, 60 seconds long, arranged from January 1st to December 31st, a prayer to each page, *written expressly for this book* by the most eminent preachers and laymen in the English-speaking world. At the top of each page is a selection of Scripture on encouragement to prayer.

Prayers by Drs. Wilfred T. Grenfell, W.W. Keen; Reverend Doctors, F.B. Meyer, John Clifford, James M. Gray, Timothy Stone, David James Burrell, Washington Gladden, Hugh Black; Rev. W. Griffith Thomas; Bishops W.A. Quayle, Charles E. Woodcock; President E.Y. Mullins, Mrs. Alice Hegan Rice, author of "Mrs. Wiggs of the Cabbage Patch." Clinton Scollard contributes an original poem.

Full cloth bound, printed on thin Rag Feather-weight paper, 384 pages. Specially priced at 60 cents a copy, cloth; in leatherette, $1.00; in art leather, $1.50.

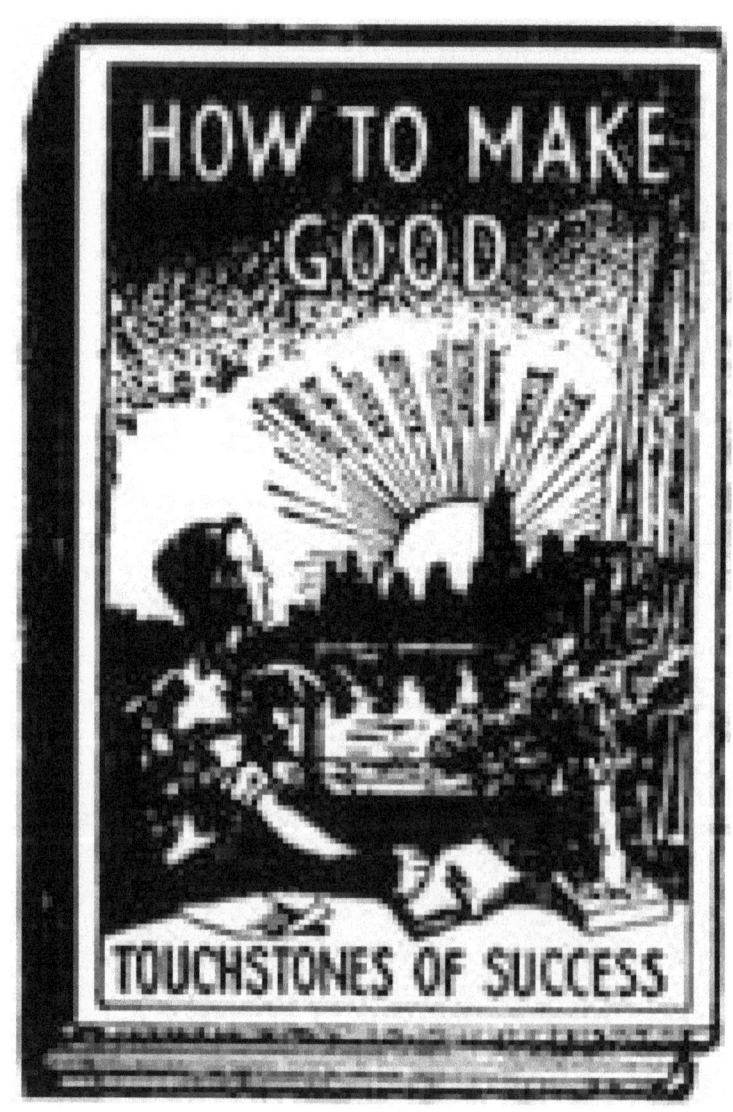

What a Young Woman Ought to Know

"Touchstones
of
Success"

WRITTEN BY

160 Present Day
Men of Achievement
Especially for
This Book

Opinions of Great Business Men

From a California National Bank: "Please find enclosed order for five copies of 'Touchstones of Success,' which we will keep in the bank for the present and future young men to read at their leisure time at the expense of the bank."

From a Widely Known California Engineer: "I enclose check for $10.00 for eight copies of Touchstones of Success'."

From a Big Business Man, Boston, Mass: "This is a splendid book for young men and it ought to be of great value to them."

From a Prominent Manufacturer in Detroit: "Please send six copies of the book. I want to distribute them among some of the employees in our office."

From a Great Manufacturing Concern of St. Louis: "I am passing copies of the book among the boys in our office because it contains some wonderful messages."

From a Widely Known New York Jurist: "I am enclosing my check for $25.00, which makes $50.00 that I have invested in extra copies of this book, so you know what I think of it."

Price, full cloth Bound, $1.25 net per copy

What a Young Woman Ought to Know

THE PUBLISHERS:
The VIR PUBLISHING COMPANY
200-214: NORTH 15TH STREET, PHILADELPHIA, PA.

A Book About Our Wonderful Bodies

Marvels of Our Bodily
Dwelling

By MRS. MARY WOOD-ALLEN, M.D.

Author of "What a Young Girl Ought
to Know," etc.

Introduction by SYLVANUS STALL. D.D.

In the form of an allegory—comparing each part of the human body to its counterpart in a dwelling, the author has succeeded in making this human study as interesting as a Sherlock Holmes detective story. She has laid under contribution the best scientific authorities and this book will be found abreast of the Science of today.

Cloth with cover in four colors, stamped in gold. 328 pages with fine half-tone pictures and 72 line drawings.

A Marvelous Book Upon a Marvelous Subject

THE VIR PUBLISHING COMPANY
PHILADELPHIA. PA., U.S.A.: 200 N. 15th Street
LONDON: 7, Imperial Arcade, Ludgate Circus, E.C.
TORONTO: Ryerson Press, 29 Richmond Street. W.

What a Young Woman Ought to Know

Bible Selections for Daily Devotion

Selected and Arranged by

SYLVANUS STALL, D.D.

This book brings to family worship 365 passages best suited in character and length to such service.

It is intended to relieve the father or mother of perplexity and apprehension concerning the passages to be read, and to enable them to bring to the service that frame of mind indispensable to the conduct of real worship.

The Gospel narrative is chronologically arranged.

The text is from the Authorized version, while the verses are merged into paragraphs as in the Revised edition.

Difficult words are pronounced.

The selections are suited not only for use in family worship, but for the chapel service of colleges, universities, and by teachers in the opening services of public schools.

Readings are from three to five minutes in length.

Lightning Source UK Ltd.
Milton Keynes UK
UKHW010634100621
385271UK00001B/65